Natural Approaches to Women's Health

Dorena Rode

Disclaimer: The information in this book is intended for educational purposes only and should not be substituted for professional medical care. Consult your health care practitioner and other resources before you adopt any wellness program since your individual constitution, state of health, and other personal factors can influences how herbs, supplements and life-style changes may affect you. The information presented is considered accurate based on the author's experience, but it may not be true for you.

Cover photo: *Vitex agnus-castus*, Experimental College Garden, UC Davis. Copyright © 2000 Dorena Rode

Rode, Dorena, 1964-
Natural approaches to Women's Health/Dorena Rode

ISBN: 1941894070
ISBN-13: 978-1941894071

1. Women's Health 2. Complementary and Alternative Medicine 3. Physiology

ȒTESLȊ
The Enlightenment & Simple Living Institute
TESLI.org

DEDICATION

To everyone who would like to have optimal health.

May the merit from this project
contribute to the sustenance of the earth
and promote optimal health for all.

ACKNOWLEDGEMENTS

I learned the western constitutional approach to herbal medicine described in this book from Adam Seller, the founder of the Pacific School of Herbal Medicine. The materia medica was prepared predominately using notes from my studies with him while incorporating my own experience. I am grateful for the additional notes provided by John Douthitt, another student of Adam's.

The cross reference list was taken from *Herbal Tinctures in Clinical Practice* (1996) by Michael Moore. I also drew heavily from Michael Moore's texts in reporting contraindications and confirming dosages and indications.

I have included Dr. Lois Johnson's recommendations for more natural hormone replacement therapies in the HRT section (pg 44). I think women will find the alternatives she recommends valuable, especially if the herbal approaches are not cutting it. In addition, I give her recipe for "cool stuff for hot women," one of my favorite combinations for hot flashes (pg 48).

TABLE OF CONTENTS

INTRODUCTION

<u>My Background</u>

I have been a plant lover from childhood. One of the first books I got when I left home at 15 years of age was *Jeanne Rose's Herbal*. I read it so many times it wore out completely. In college I took a folk medicine class that introduced me to many healing modalities. As a result of that class I enrolled in a practitioner's course in Traditional Chinese Medicine when I was 17 years old. In the two year practitioner course I learned the diagnostic system of Chinese Medicine, an extensive materia medica, the five element theory, and how to work with the body as an integrated whole. Also in college, my copy of Mrs. M. Grieves' *A Modern Herbal* allowed me to take the handout on weeds from my horticulture class and identify the medicinal or nutritional properties of each plant. It amazed me how we ignored the potential food and medicine volunteering around us freely. As I preferred Western herbs to herbs imported from China, I began studying the plants that grew around my home in California. Concurrently, I studied natural product chemistry at UCSC and earned my bachelor's degree in chemistry with highest honors.

Over the next decade I went out into the work world, got married, had a daughter and got divorced. It was during the divorce transition that I began to rekindle my love of herbal medicine. I studied with Adam Seller at the Pacific School of Herbal Medicine. He used an western constitutional approach to herbal medicine. It was the closet I'd seen to a system like Chinese medicine. However, it utilized our western physiology and our western plants. I was so excited by the system he presented that I returned to school and earned a doctorate in physiology. My research was funded by the National Institute of Health - National Center for Alternative and Complementary Medicine (NIH-NCCAM). I investigated the effects of herbs and stress on female reproductive hormones.

During this time, I began to be fascinated by the placebo effect. It seemed to me that if the mind was so powerful, why not work directly with the mind. Herbs and drugs did not work all the time. What was up with that? I envisioned a new medical system that would put the mind at the center of the equation.

After I graduated I did some post-doctoral work with researchers at Kaiser and also attempted to pursue a post-doctoral program at UCSF. I was invited to interview, but it turned out they wanted me to continue with my herbal research, while I wanted to explore the effects that energy or mental modalities had on health. In particular, I was interested in studying ThetaHealing® a method I had learned for accessing and changing limiting beliefs. I had such dramatic results using the ThetaHealing technique on myself and clients; I was curious about finding a way to demonstrate its efficacy.

This marked my entry in to a period where external prospects seemed to completely dry up. The next decade marked an intense period of internal exploration and expansion. The majority of my time was spent in meditation, practicing internal arts and healing from childhood trauma that I had repressed. I slowly transitioned out of my cocoon and 2015 marked my formal emergence.

Objectives

The information I present here is a combination of ancient wisdom, modern science, and new age thought. My objective is to provide you with an understanding of how the body functions on a physical level and explain how to use herbs, foods, and supplements to balance your body's hormones and systems related to women's health. I will also touch on how our thoughts, experiences, and subconscious beliefs influence our energy bodies and how those in turn affect our physical body. Not everything I say will ring true for you. Take what you like and leave the rest.

Disclaimer

The information in this book is intended for educational purposes only and should not be substituted for professional medical care. Consult your health care practitioner and other resources before you adopt any wellness program since your individual constitution, state of health, and other personal factors can influences how herbs, supplements and life-style changes may affect you. The information presented is considered accurate based on my experience, but it may not be true for you.

For instance, nettles is a common nutritive herb and food. Indeed, in Britain it is sold as cream of nettles soup. In United States and United Kingdom it is considered to be completely safe to use in any quantity. It really is a food and many women use it during pregnancy because it is rich in minerals. The fresh plant is also a potent anti-histamine and perfect for allergies. I once recommended it to a pregnant friend with hay fever. She was early in her pregnancy and started having uterine cramping/contractions. Thanks to the internet, I was able to find out that nettles does have this effect on Indian women but not on Caucasians.

Make sure you check with your inner knowing before you make any health decision. It is also good to follow up with an internet search, to see if new or unusual reports are available.

Best of health!

SCIENTIFIC VALIDATION

In the last decade or two there has been a lot of emphasis on evidence-based practices. My opinion on this focus can be best summed up by Simon Mills (a medical herbalist): "...perhaps the fact that 90% of all scientists in history are alive today is a reflection of an age out of touch with itself."

Operating within the construct that the only reasonable drug, herb or practice to use is one that has been validated scientifically is an incredible limitation for a number of reasons.

1) Lack of Research

First imagine everything that exists. For this example I will depict "everything", including the entirety of knowledge, as a circle.

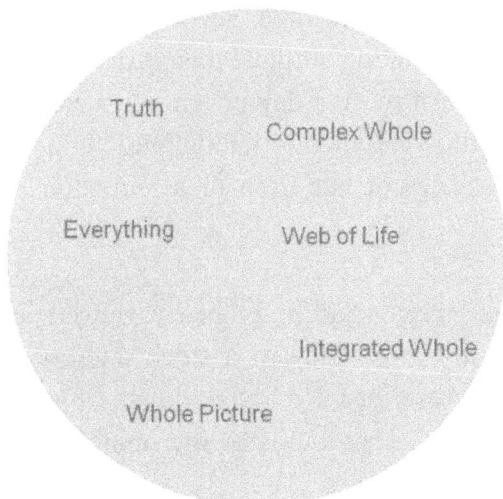

Truth

Complex Whole

Everything

Web of Life

Integrated Whole

Whole Picture

In the next picture, the black dots on the circle represent our present day scientific knowledge. Actually, this is probably an exaggeration, we know much less, but I wanted you to be able to see the dots. The number one limitation of basing what herb or drug to choose on scientific knowledge is the extreme lack of knowledge we have. In addition, notice how spread out the dots are. We know a little bit about a wide range of topics, but we don't have a complete picture of the integrated whole.

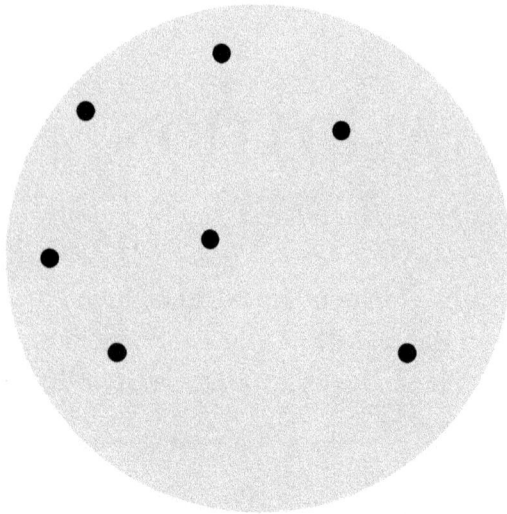

I personally have found very few research studies that reflect what would truly inform actual clinical practice. It is too hard and too limiting to do a study that reflects reality. Reality is too complex, so studies are designed to be simple and only ask a simple question.

Not only does the question need to be simple, it needs to be specific. For instance, "Does *Cimicifuga* (black cohosh) reduce hot flashes?" is too general. First, the type of extract of *Cimicifuga* needs to be specified and a complete chemical profile performed. Second, the dosing needs to be specified. Third, what is the population? Are we talking surgical menopause? Are we talking natural menopause. Do the women have a hot flash twice a day or ten times a day? Other considerations are the women's ethnicity, culture, lifestyle, dietary habits, etc. Fourth, what do we consider a reduction? Will this be less instances of hot flash or a reduction in intensity? How do you measure intensity?

Studies that reflect clinically relevant question are rare. For instance, I once reviewed an excellent study on irritable bowel syndrome that compared the efficacy of a stock traditional Chinese herbal formula with a custom blended formula prescribed by a traditional Chinese medical doctor. The doctor did better than the stock formula. That validated my opinion that herbs need to matched to people, not disease names, so I liked the study.

What were the limitations of the study? Well, maybe that doctor just happened to be better than your typical doctor. Indeed, the study really only validated the one doctor, but not the idea that custom formulation based on an individual's constitution is better. In addition, scientifically, no conclusion is considered valid unless it can be replicated by another independent researcher. This study was not repeated, as is common with herbal research. Who's going to pay for a study that cannot be used to make a profit?

2) Research Flaws

Flawed research is really an extension of what I was just writing about. It is important to consider research flaws, because if the research used as the basis of an evidence-based practice is flawed, then people are not getting the highest quality of care. Scientifically, there is not a study out there that is flawless. Indeed, researchers get together weekly, review other people's work, and discuss the limitations (which is an nice way of saying they tear the research apart).

Actually one of the most flawed scientific designs from a practical perspective is what is considered the gold standard of clinical research: the double-blind, randomized, placebo-controlled study. The assumption behind this research design is that substances have inherent power and efficacy and that people's opinions, attitudes, beliefs, expectations, and intentions also have power. This research is designed to tease apart the inherent power of the drug from the inherent power of the mind. This is a worthy goal, but this research tends to devalue the mind's power and suggest a substance's power is more real or valid. Indeed, the placebo effect is often eluded to as an effect that is not really real or worthy of notice.

Personally, I do not understand why, once the placebo effect was recognized, researchers didn't focus more on optimizing the inherent healing ability of the mind. If the mind is so powerful, why are we even bothering with drugs? I suppose this may have something to do with the economics of selling drugs. In addition, this type of research is just a left-over from the limiting worldview based on Newtonian physics. In Newtonian physics a drug has an action and will always produce a predictable effect. This is a comfortable idea for many people. Quantum physics supports the idea that a wide range of possibilities are possible and that we, as humans, can influence the outcome of a drug's effect. Explaining the world as cause and effect will eventually fall by the wayside, along with double-blind, placebo-controlled studies, as our society adopts a worldview more in alignment with quantum physics.

What is the greatest limitation of research that is based on the double-blind, randomized, placebo-controlled study? Well, it is possible that some substances are more active when combined with the mind. This important interaction is neglected in a study designed to take all human connection and intention out of the picture. Further, human variation is amazing. It is possible that people will gravitate to the right treatment for their health problem and the idea of randomly assigning them to a test group limits the broad applicability of the results. A treatment that "doesn't work" with the population tested, may actually be the perfect cure for certain individuals that might naturally seek out that treatment.

Other common flaws in herbal research are:

Dosing does not reflect clinical practice. I've seen this in research on herbs versus the common cold. I, personally, can stop any cold using *Berberis*. The key things are starting at first onset of cold symptoms and using high and frequent doses as needed to stop symptom progression. If I start when I just feel tired, I just need a squirt or two of tincture every once and awhile. If I start after my throat feels sore, I need a squirt of tincture every half hour until my throat doesn't feel sore, then I can cut back.

Research was done on a single herb that is usually used in combination. Or vice versa, the research tests a proprietary blend. I was taught that herbs are feeble, but that the target effect of a combination of herbs can have a bigger impact. Still, many herbs are tested using the drug model that ignores the synergistic effects of herbal combinations.

Research was done on a form of the plant not usually used clinically. Often times companies want to validate their product and they fund research on their preparation. It is common to assume that all preparations of the plant will work similarly, but that is just an assumption. It is also assumed that each batch of the plant will work similarly, but because of natural product variability, you cannot even count on that.

Natural products and extraction methods are variable. This is not really a flaw in the research, but does represent a limitation of using research reports about herbs. I used to get menstrual migraines. I was using an alcohol extract of feverfew to reduce the frequency and intensity of those headaches. It seemed to be working. Then some research was released that demonstrated that the powered herb was effective, but not an alcohol extract. I believed it and stopped using the tincture. My headaches got worse. When I resumed taking the extract I once again experience fewer headaches with milder intensity.

Botanical product not characterized. Much of the older herb research doesn't even report if they confirmed they had the right plant or the correct part of the plant (root vs. leaf vs. seed, etc). Sorry, scientists make the assumption if they buy something it actually is what they think it is, but herbs are not as straightforward as chemicals. They may also neglect to explain how the plant was extracted. In addition, the chemical analysis of the plant, which is critical to determining if one batch is equivalent to another, is rarely done or reported. Again, there was an assumption that natural products have no variability.

A traditionally used herbs was tested out of context. When herbs are used as part of traditional healing systems other components, such as ritual and/or song, may be necessary to activate the herb. For instance, in Tibetan Buddhism there are mixtures of herbs that allow meditative practitioners to go for long periods of time without food. These herbs have to be activated by special words (mantras) and are used in conjunction with specific practices.

Test subjects do not match you. The results of using an herb may differ based on the person's lifestyle, diet, ethnicity, etc. For instance, nettles is a common nutritive herb and food. Indeed, in Britain it is sold as cream of nettles soup. In United States and United Kingdom it is considered to be completely safe to use in any quantity. It really is a food and many women use it during pregnancy because it is rich in minerals. The fresh plant is also a potent anti-histamine and perfect for allergies. I once recommended it to a pregnant friend with hay fever. She was early in her pregnancy and started having uterine cramping/contractions. Thanks to the internet, I was able to find out that nettles does have this effect on Indian women.

Delivery method is not traditional. Some of the research coming out of Europe, where use of herbs is a standard practice in medicine, uses injectable herbal extracts. The results of using an injectable form may not reflect what the herb does if taken orally. One example is the treatment of Amanita mushroom poisoning using a milk thistle extract intravenously. In the United States, mushroom poisoning is treated with liver transplants. We don't have the IV extract they have in Europe and the oral preparations will not protect a liver from Amanita mushroom poisoning. (If you are going to eat poisonous mushrooms, better do it in Europe. Think about the differences in cost and human suffering!)

Placebo used was not really inactive. It is hard to find an inert substance to match a strong tasting herb for a placebo controlled study. I've seen research on the common cold that used alfalfa as the placebo. Apparently the researchers didn't know that alfalfa is an herb that is used in the treatment of the common cold. It's not a primary defense, but it does support the body's ability to carry waste out of the body.

Subjects can figure out if they have the placebo or herb. If the researchers pick something that is really just filler, many people can figure out they don't have the active substance and the study is not longer "blind". When I was at UC Davis a women enrolled in a long term study involving gingko and the prevention of Alzheimer's called me. She was worried about developing the disease and did not want to spend years on the placebo. I told her to just open the capsule and taste the contents. It did have flavor, but she wanted to be sure it was gingko so she came over. I tasted it and assured her she was getting gingko. Opps! Study no longer placebo controlled.

Confounding factors matter. Research has shown that the color of the tablet makes a difference in psychiatric medications. The timing of treatment also makes a difference. Rats undergoing radiation therapy for cancer will either live or die depending on the time of day the treatment was given due to daily fluctuations in cortisol levels. Season and stage of the lunar cycle may also be important in treatment outcome. And, of course, intention and subconscious beliefs can influence treatment results.

3) Incomplete and Inaccurate Research Reports

Let's consider the study design we were talking about earlier regarding *Cimicifuga* and hot flashes (pg 6). Perhaps someone decides to run that study and finds out that a standardized extract of *Cimicifuga* (30 mg three times a day) does not reduce the number of hot flashes in Caucasian women that have just undergone a hysterectomy. By the time the results hit the news all you learn is that the study demonstrated that *Cimicifuga* doesn't work. However, this doesn't mean that a woman undergoing natural menopause wouldn't see a reduction in hot flash intensity with using half that dose. The results of the study are interesting, but may not apply to you unless your situation is identical.

In addition, many people rely of scientific summaries or research abstracts for information. Unfortunately, these are often designed to be sensational or intriguing. Even if they are accurate, they are written with a world limit and a lot of information has to be left out. I have found that upon reading the full article the results are not really as clinically relevant as the abstract would lead one to believe.

Why don't people read the full article? It is an access issue. Researchers and students have access to the full scientific reports as part of their institutional perk. For private individuals one article can sometimes cost more than $30. There has been a shift in recent years to require research done with public funds to be accessible to the public, but it doesn't really solve the problem of restricted access to other research. Hard to make an educated decision when you are unable to get access to the full report.

4) Research Bias

The results of research can be distorted based on conflicts of interest. The most common conflict of interest is when researchers have a financial investment in the research showing a positive result. The most obvious form of this is when the researcher is testing a product or service that they sell personally or they own stock or interest in a company that does. This conflict of interest would include a relative or friend selling the product they are testing. In that case they would have an *interest* in the success of their relative or friend.

Although, researchers are supposed to indicate any conflict of interest, they may want to present their interest as unbiased and will neglect to mention any conflict of interest that is not a direct financial gain. Indeed, sometimes the funding agency is a foundation that upon closer inspection appears to have been set up so that a researcher can launder the financial contribution to the study by having the funding come from the foundation rather than directly from the manufacturer of the test preparation.

Direct financial gain isn't the only way researchers may make money on studies. Many researchers need to publish interesting research in order to maintain their careers and ensure future research funds. Researchers make a living by getting someone to fund their research. An interesting research proposal will gain funding, but a researcher needs to report satisfactory progress each year to maintain that funding. A researcher may feel pressure to make a study work. I once heard a statistician say, "If you think there is an effect, we can find a way to make the statistics show it."

In addition, researcher may be motivated by fame or just wanting to be right. Once I talked to a former student that worked for a researcher who had her run chemical analysis on samples over and over until, by a fluke, the data matched the researcher's hypothesis. The researcher would review the data and circle the samples to rerun. The student reported that the repeated samples would give the same result, but researcher would have her rerun them over and over. Eventually, a run would give the value that fit with what the researcher wanted. The student could see the farce in this, but as long as the researcher had an actual result, they did not feel like they were falsifying data.

5) Pharmaceutical Research

We've been talking about research that is what I might call "pure" research. Pharmaceutical drugs studies actually fall outside of traditional scientific research channels, so it is best to consider them separately.

Pharmaceutical companies are interested in getting their product okayed by the FDA as a drug. They develop the drug, pay for the studies, and run the studies themselves in conjunction with medical test sites. Their research is inherently biased. The people running the studies are paid by the pharmaceutical company. The data they collect is prepared in house and submitted to the FDA for approval. There is no peer review process where the data is evaluated before publication. Publication of the research is not the objective, the objective is to demonstrate the safety of the drug and that it can be used to treat a certain disease. They are focused on "selling" their drug to the FDA so they can get it on the market. There is an assumption that they are not falsifying data.

Another bias is present in the FDA review process itself. Members of FDA advisory panels are allowed to have financial ties to drug companies and still participate in the approval process.[1] For example, in recent years the contraceptive drugs Yaz and Yasim were implicated in 100 deaths, demonstrated a three-fold increase in blood clot risk, and 12,000 unhappy patients were suing for damages. The FDA finally decided to investigate the drugs. The advisory panel voted 15 to 11 to keep the drugs on the market. Four or five of the panel members had financial interests in the company that produced the drugs. They were all allowed to vote and voted to keep the drug on the market. Another doctor, that had written an article calling for the drugs to be removed from the market, was kicked off the panel for an "intellectual conflict of interest".

In addition to bias within the advisory panel, it is not uncommon for the FDA staff to have worked in the industry they will be regulating as part of the FDA. Further, key policy makers may also have financial ties to the industry they regulate.

In addition, sometimes drug studies come up with a significant effect that is clinically irrelevant. A hypothetical example might be a drug that significantly reduces cholesterol. That sounds really good until you look at the clinical reality that the drug has a bunch of side effects and the reduction of cholesterol was only 1%. This means if someone has a high cholesterol value of 245 the drug would bring it down to 243. The reduction is actually meaningless and the patient still has high cholesterol.

You might wonder, would a doctor actually prescribe a drug that was so worthless. Maybe. Doctors receive their drug education along with gifts, free samples, and perks from drug companies. They would be told the hypothetical drug is FDA approved for the reduction of cholesterol. Why would they question it further?

The hypothetical situation demonstrates how this might work, but this is exactly what is going on with anti-depressants. It has long been know that anti-depressants work just as well as placebo in patients with mild, moderate and even severe depression. Indeed, they only show true clinical efficacy in patients that are very severely depressed.[2] Yet, doctors still prescribe them. They are expensive placebos with unpleasant side effects.

KEY TERMS

Key Terms

This is a glossary of terms used in the text. I put it at the front because I wanted you to know it is here as a reference, not because I think you should read it. Feel free to skim through it for fun and return to it if you want more information about a term.

adaptogens

Adaptogens recalibrate the body's systems, i.e. if blood pressure is high, they bring it down. If blood pressure is low, they bring it up. If thyroid is low, they elevate it. If thyroid is high, they bring it down. Examples: Eleutherococcus (Siberian Ginseng), Withania (Ashwagandha), Ganoderma (Reishi).

allopathic medicine

The system of medical practice which treats disease by the use of remedies which produce effects different from those produced by the disease under treatment. This is the way mainstream medical doctors operate.

anterior pituitary

Endocrine organ in the head that secretes a wide variety of hormones: ACTH, TSH, LH, FSH, PRL, GH, and MSH.

cervix

The lower section of the uterus that surrounds a narrow canal that opens into the vagina.

clitoris

Erectile tissue that is at the top of the vulva. It is homologous to the penis.

corpus albicans

Literally it means white (albicans) body (corpus). Fibrous tissue that remains after a corpus luteum decays.

corpus luteum

Literally it means yellow (luteum) body (corpus). The cells of the follicle after ovulation are transformed into this yellow tissue that produces progesterone. If the ovum is not fertilized it decays into the corpus albicans.

endocrine

Of or related to cells, tissue, glands or organs that secrete hormones directly into the bloodstream.

fallopian tube

A tube that extends from the ovary to the uterus in which the ova pass. Also know as oviduct.

FSH (follicle stimulating hormone)

Hormone released by the anterior pituitary. Its main target is follicular cells of ovary. It stimulates the growth of the follicle and the production of estrogen.

Follicle

An ovarian follicle includes the oocyte and the cells that surround the oocyte. There are several developmental phases of a follicle:

- A primordial follicle is dormant and small with one layer of granulosa cells surrounding the oocyte.
- A primary follicle is active and growing. It has one layer of granulosa cells.
- A secondary follicle has multiple layers of granulosa cells and surrounding those are thecal cells.
- An antral follicle has a fluid filled center. One layer of granulosa cells surrounds the oocyte and more granulosa cells surround the antrum (the fluid filled center). Thecal cells surround all that. The antral follicle is ten times larger than the secondary follicle.
- In the graafian follicle the antrum is larger. The width of the follicle is ten times that of the antral follicle. It measure about 10 to 20 mm across.

Genitals

External sex organs. In the female these are also called the vulva.

Gonad
The organs (testes or ovaries) that produce gametes (sperm or ovum).

GnRH (gonadotropin releasing hormone)
Hormone formed in the hypothalamus that stimulates the release of FSH and LH by the anterior pituitary.

hormones
Chemicals produced by one tissue (typically endocrine glands or neurons) that travel in the bloodstream to activate/deactivate a target tissue that can be the same or different than the producing tissue. These are also considered chemical messengers or regulatory substances.

hypothalamus
An area of the brain that coordinates both the autonomic nervous system and the activity of the pituitary. It is made of various neural centers with specialized function such as controlling body temperature, thirst, hunger, and other homeostatic systems as well as sleep and emotional activity. Because of its regulation of the pituitary, it is considered a bridge between the nervous system and the endocrine system.

LH (luteinizing hormone).
A hormone produced by the anterior pituitary. Its main target is the follicular cells in the ovary. It stimulates the production of the precursor to estrogen in the developing follicle. A surge in LH induces ovulation. After ovulation it stimulates the production of progesterone by the corpus luteum.

Menopause
Menopause is, strictly speaking, the date when your menses have stopped permanently. This is calculated backwards after you've gone for one year without a period. Natural menopause usually occurs between 45 to 55 years of age. The time period after menopause is referred to as postmenopausal while the time period just prior to menopause is referred to as perimenopausal.

menstruation
A women's monthly discharge of blood and mucosal tissue from the uterus. Also known as period or menses.

menstrual cycle

A monthly cycle of uterine and ovarian changes that make pregnancy possible. If pregnancy does not occur menstruation (the sloughing of the uterine lining) occurs and the cycle begins again.

neurons

Cells that release chemicals that regulate the body's activities. Neurons secrete either neurotransmitters or hormones. Both neurotransmitters and hormones are chemical messengers. Neurotransmitters travel a short distance to their target (typically the next neuron, a muscle or a gland), while hormones travel longer distance via the bloodstream.

neural centers or nuclei

A group of specialized neurons in the brain that are packed together. They can be identified functionally and/or visibly. Important neural centers in the hypothalamus are the medial preoptic nucleus which produces GnRH, the supraoptic nucleus that produces oxytocin, and the anterior hypothalamic nucleus that is involved in thermoregulation.

ovary

An organ that produces the ova, eggs, or sex cells. Ovaries are homologous with testes.

ovum (plural - ova)

The egg, gamete, or sex cell.

oxytocin

A hormone released from the posterior pituitary. It participates in uterine contractions, orgasmic contractions, and the let down of milk during lactation.

Perimenopause

Perimenopause is the time leading up to menopause and is characterized by menstrual irregularities as well as emotional and hormonal fluctuations. Since the normal menstrual cycle is characterized by hormonal fluctuations many of the complaints women have regarding the perimenopausal period can be addressed in the same manner as the similar complaints experienced by women in their twenties, thirties and early forties.

posterior pituitary

The terminal ends of hypothalamic neurons form the posterior pituitary. These neurons release the hormones oxytocin and vasopressin.

PRL (prolactin)

A hormone produced by the anterior pituitary. Prolactin stimulates the development of breast tissue and the production of milk during lactation. Prolactin levels are increased with stress and after orgasm. Prolactin inhibits the release of GnRH.

systemic circulation

The general blood circulation of the body.

uterus

The organ that receives the fertilized ovum and holds the developing fetus. The uterus is homologous with the prostrate.

vagina

Muscular tissue that forms the passage way between the external genitalia and the uterus.

vulva

Female external sex organs or genitalia. Includes labia, clitoris, and opening to the urethra.

THE REPRODUCTIVE SYSTEM

Before we get into the details of what is going on during a woman's menstrual cycle, lets first introduce the important players. Feel free to look up any unfamiliar terms in the previous chapter. For this discussion we will consider a woman during the years she is actively menstruating. This is just a quick overview. We will get into the details later.

The main controllers of the reproductive organs are located in the head. The hypothalamus contains neural centers that release hormones that travel a short distance by a special blood supply to the anterior pituitary. There the hypothalamic hormones activate the endocrine tissue to release hormones that enter the systemic circulation. The hypothalamus also contains specialized neurons that extend down to the posterior pituitary where they release hormones directly into systemic circulation.

Hormones from the pituitary travel in the blood supply and bind to receptors on the follicular cells in the ovaries. In response, these cells produce estrogen and the follicles grow. The follicles contain the oocytes. Each normal cycle one follicle will reach complete maturation and release a secondary oocyte. In the ovary, those follicular cells will be transformed into the corpus luteum which produces progesterone. Progesterone is a hormone that tells the uterus to hang onto that rich menstrual lining in case the egg is fertilized.

Meanwhile, the egg floats down the fallopian tube propelled by a gentle current created by the cilia on the lining of fallopian tube. If fertilization does not occur in the fallopian tube, the ovum only lives about 24 hours. About two weeks after ovulation the corpus luteum degrades and the uterus sheds the lining.

If fertilization does occur, an event that requires more than 40 million sperm deposited in the vagina, cell division begins immediately and the fertilized egg (called a blastocyst at this stage) attaches to the lining of the uterus. The blastocyst implants six to nine days after ovulation.

Figure 3: Reproductive hormone cascade.

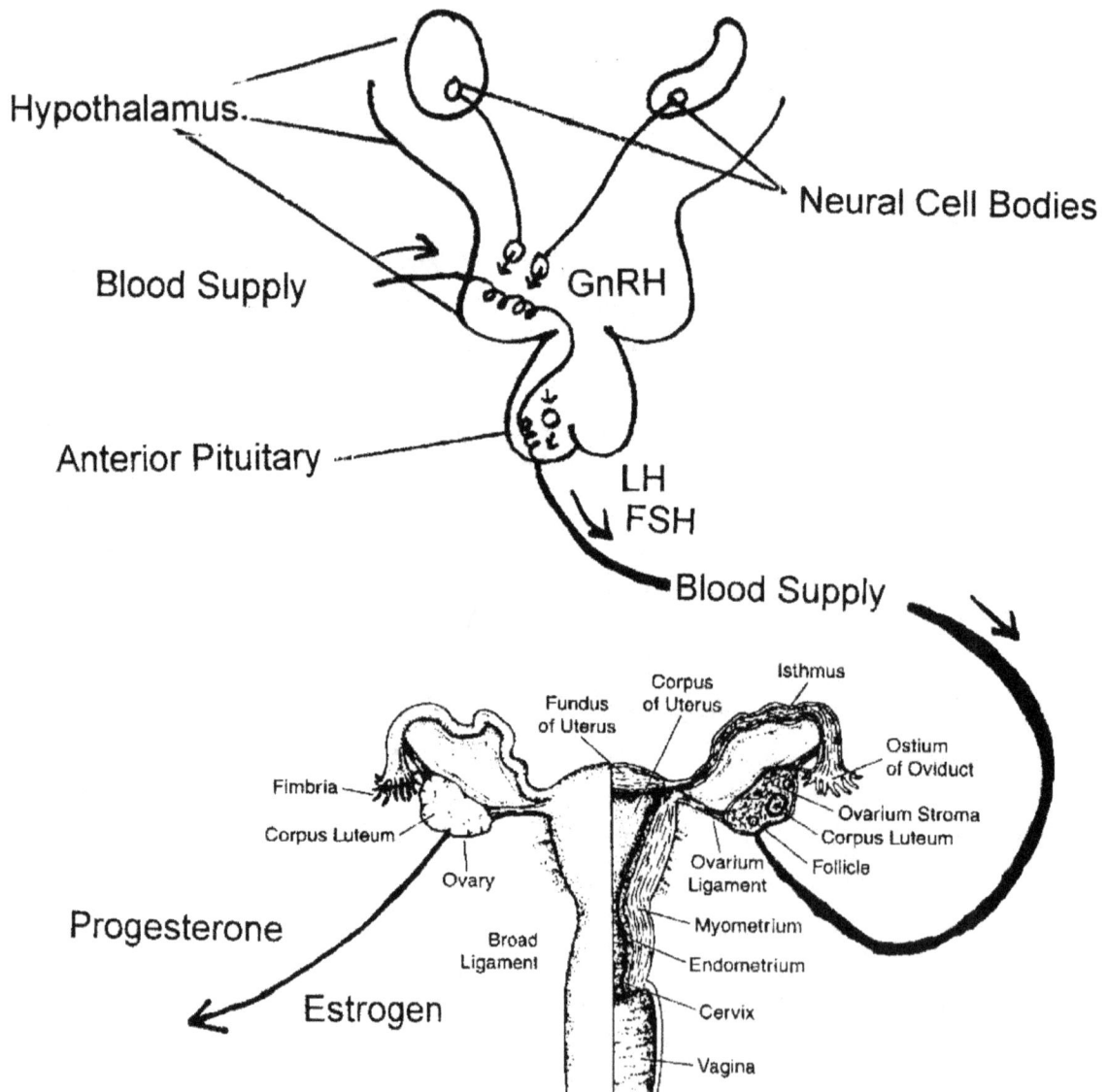

Figure 4: Important structures of the female reproductive system.

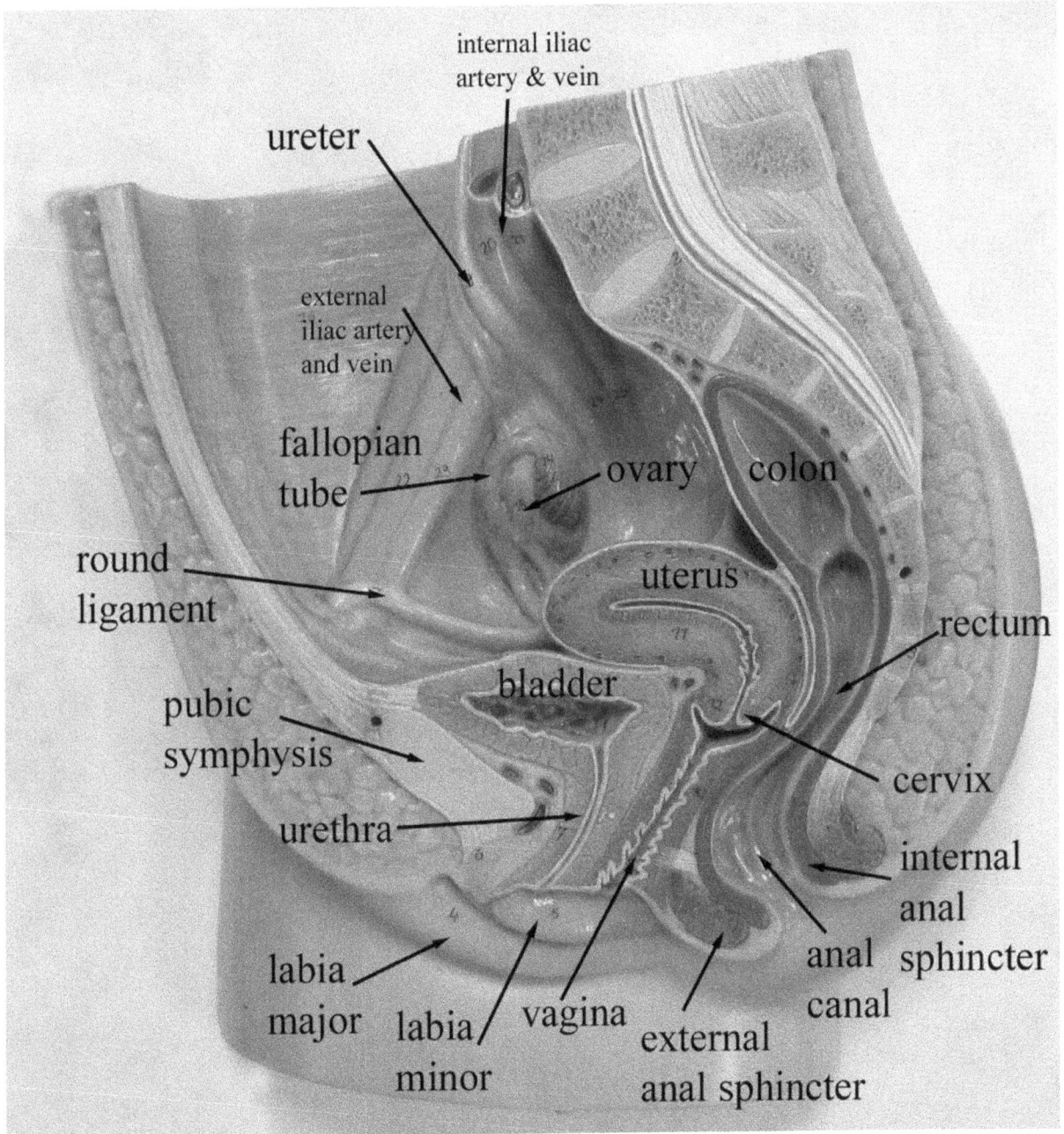

internal iliac artery & vein

ureter

external iliac artery and vein

fallopian tube

ovary

colon

round ligament

uterus

rectum

pubic symphysis

bladder

urethra

cervix

internal anal sphincter

labia major

labia minor

vagina

external anal sphincter

anal canal

Figure 5: Important structures in the ovary

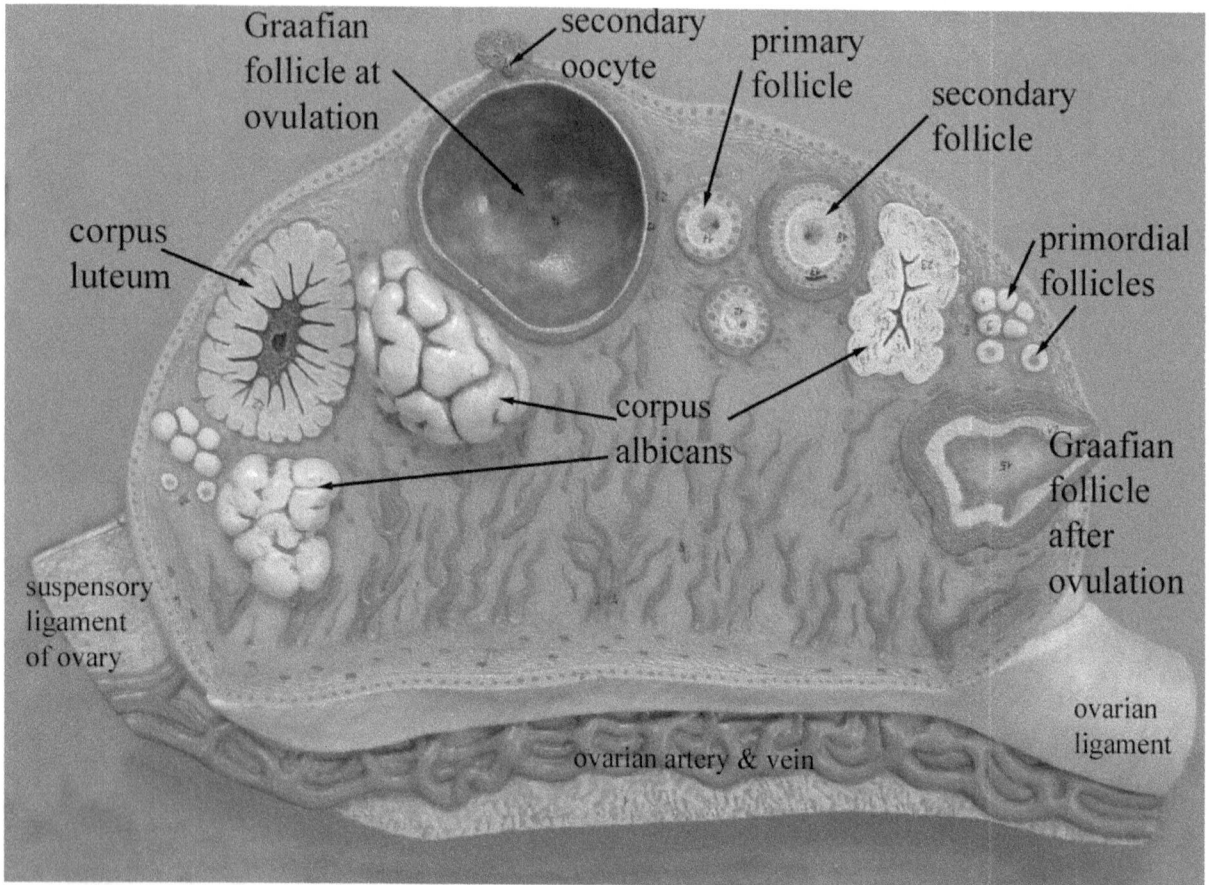

Figure 6: Histology of the ovary

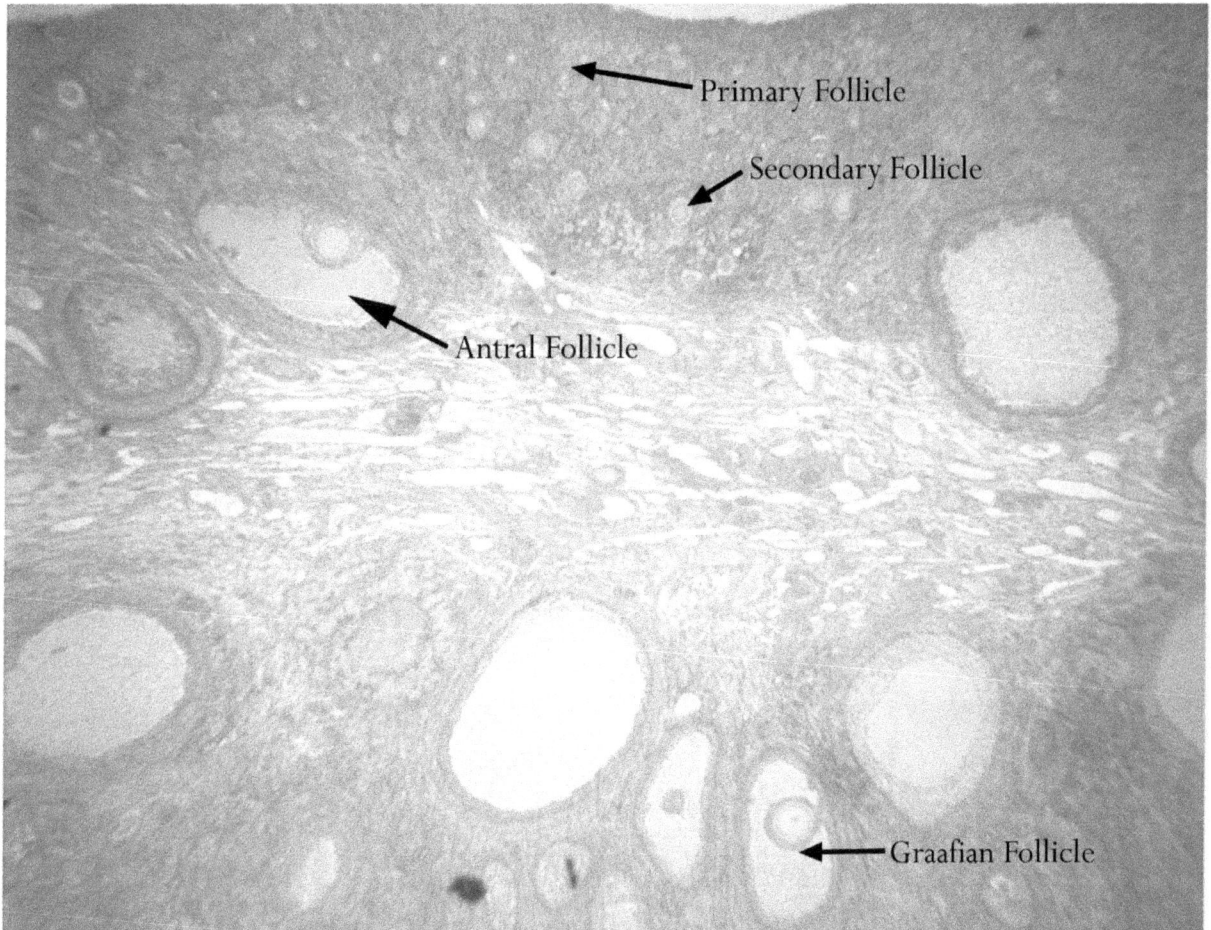

Figure 7: How the body synthesizes estrogens and progesterone from cholesterol.
This illustrates how structurally similar all the steroid hormones are. Notice how cortisol is synthesized from progesterone and how testosterone is the precursor of estrogen.

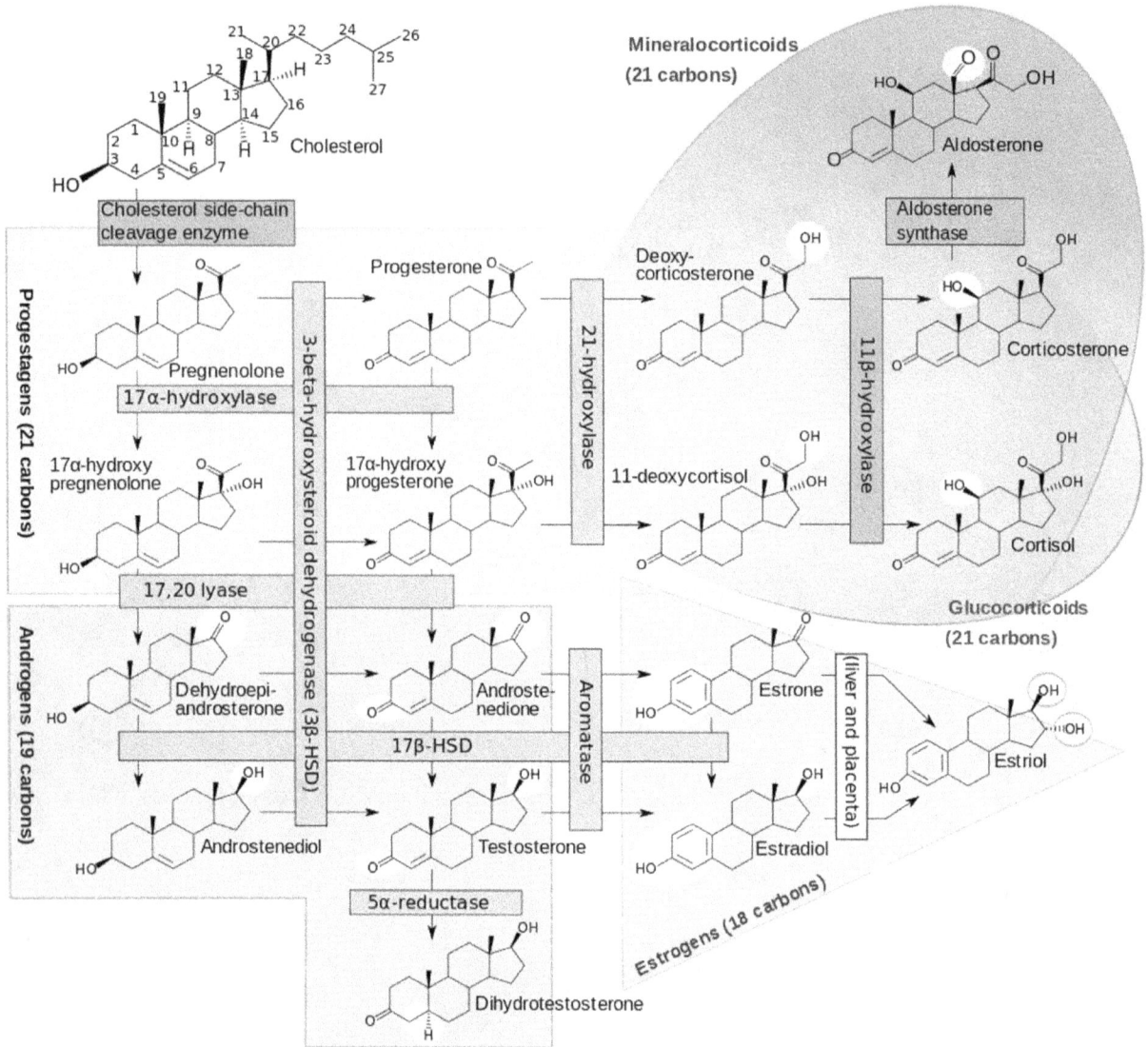

Illustration courtesy of Wikipedia: Häggström M, Richfield D (2014). "Diagram of the pathways of human steroidogenesis". Wikiversity Journal of Medicine 1 (1). DOI: 10.15347/wjm/2014.005. ISSN 20018762.

A WOMEN'S MONTHLY CYCLE

The Reproductive Time Line

A newborn girl has all the eggs (oocytes) she will ever have when she is born: about two million. (Contrast this to the male that makes fresh spermatozoa on a daily basis.) Each egg is surrounded by specialized cells and a layer of matrix that the cells produce. Collectively the oocyte, the matrix and the surrounding cells are called a follicle. Throughout childhood, on an ongoing basis, some of the follicles begin to mature. However, this process is arrested at an early stage and the eggs die off. Primordial (dormant) follicles can develop into primary and secondary follicles without additional hormonal support, but further development requires hormones (figure 8). By the time a female reaches puberty she has only 400,000 eggs and follicles left.

Beginning in puberty neurons in the hypothalamus secretes gonadotropin releasing hormone (GnRH) which stimulates the anterior pituitary to release luteinizing hormone (LH) and follicle stimulating hormone (FSH). The two gonadotropins, LH and FSH, travel in the blood to target cells in the ovary.

LH stimulates some of the follicular cells to produce an estrogen precursor. FSH acts in a synergistic manner to complete the production of estrogen. Then together FSH and estrogen stimulate the further

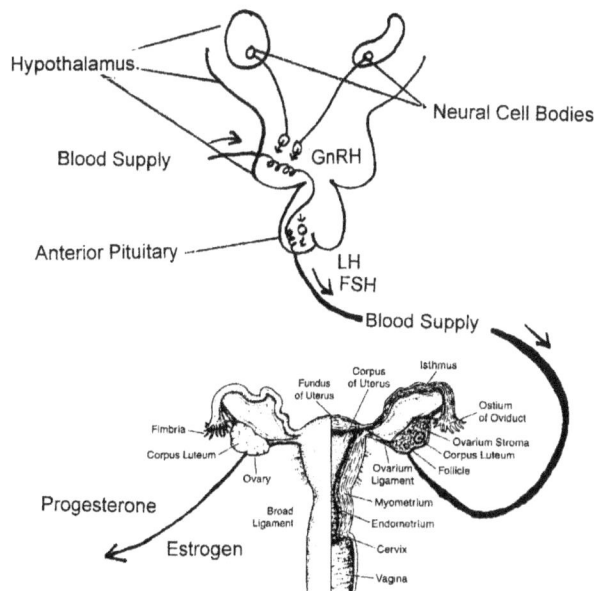

development of the follicles. Ovulation occurs when one follicle matures and releases the egg into the oviduct (fallopian tube). See figure 8.

Throughout a woman's lifetime she will ovulate only about 400 oocytes. That suggests that for each egg that makes it, about 1000 others die off before they reach maturity. The exact length of time it takes for a dormant primordial follicle to reach maturity is estimated to be at least seven months and probably more like a year. This means that during any one menstrual cycle there are follicles at many different stages of development in the ovary.

Figure 8: Follicular development
Follicular development can take seven months to one year to complete.

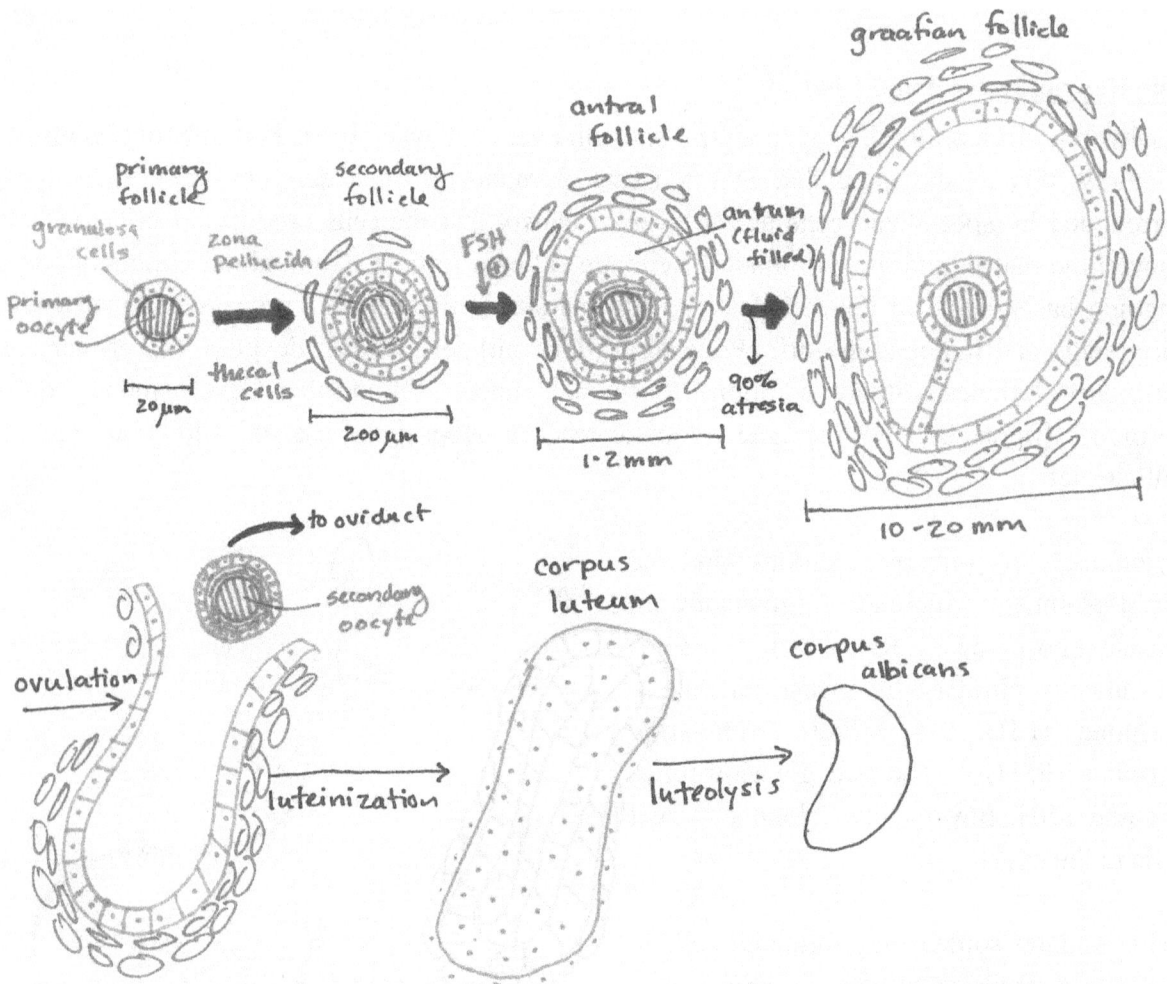

While figure 8 shows the linear development of one follicle, many follicles are developing over any one menstrual cycle and the development of any one follicle spans many menstrual cycles. This is an important factor to consider when using therapies to balance the reproductive system. If you are working to make a change using physical substances like herbs and supplements, it may take several cycles to realize results. Many women report lengthy dysregulation of their cycle when coming off birth control pills. This is probably due to the fact that follicular development has been disrupted and it may take a year for it to reestablish as normal. The time it takes to reestablish a normal cycle can be shortened using herbal approaches.

Menopause occurs as a result of simply running out of viable follicles. Without an adequate number of follicles attempting to mature each cycle the estrogen level will not be high enough to support the complete maturation of any one of them.

The Menstrual Cycle

The average menstrual cycle length is 28 days, the length of the lunar cycle. It can be divided into two distinct phases: the follicular phase and the luteal phase. From day one (first day of menstrual bleeding) until ovulation (about day 14) is the follicular phase. The luteal phase begins at ovulation and lasts until menstrual bleeding starts again (typically 14 days).

Figure 9: Hormonal fluctuations throughout the menstrual cycle

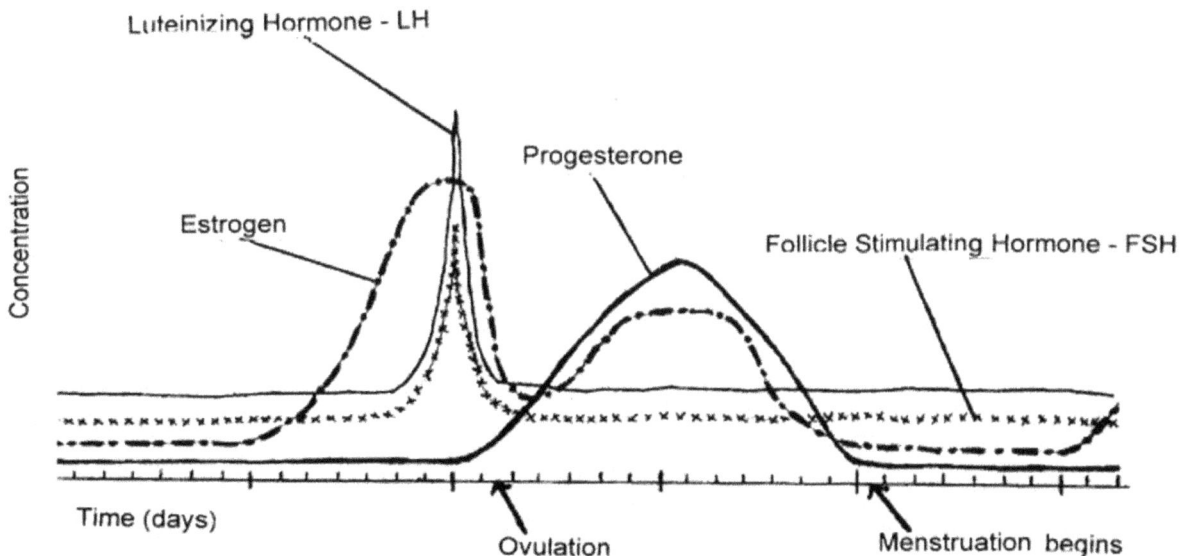

Follicular Phase

Development of follicles overlaps the menstrual cycle so that follicles begin maturing for the next cycle soon after ovulation. On day one of the menstrual cycle there are about 10 antral follicles of various sizes. These follicles are dependent on FSH for growth. Ninety percent of these will undergo atresia (die off), so by day seven one dominate follicle is left. This dominate follicle is producing a great deal of estrogen. Although levels of LH and FSH remain essentially constant throughout the menstrual cycle, this high estrogen triggers a surge of the gonadotropins at midcycle. The LH surge stimulates ovulation and luteinization. Ovulation occurs sixteen hours after the LH peak. In women who are not subject to a lot of night-time light pollution, ovulation tends to synchronize with the full moon.

Luteal Phase

The luteal phase begins at ovulation and lasts until menstrual bleeding starts again (typically 14 days). After ovulation the luteal cells (formed from the follicular cells) begin producing progesterone (and some estradiol) under the stimulus of LH and FSH. The secretion of hormones depicted in the following figure 9 is an "idealized" snapshot of one human menstrual cycle when fertilization of the ovum doesn't occur.

When the follicle releases the egg at ovulation it is transformed into a yellow body called the corpus luteum (CL). The cells of the corpus luteum produce progesterone and some estrogen. Table 1 lists some of the actions of estrogen and progesterone. Under the influence of estrogen the uterus develops and a rich lining is created for the fertilized egg to implant in. Progesterone is what maintains the uterine lining. The life span of the corpus luteum is normally 14 days. When the CL regresses at the end of the menstrual cycle the lining of the uterus is sloughed off and passes out of the body via the vagina.

TABLE 1: Estrogen and Progesterone Effects

Tissue	Physiological Action of **Estradiol**	Physiological Action of **Progesterone**
CNS	• maintains libido and sexual behavior	• inhibits LH/FSH secretion at the hypothalamus during the luteal phase
Pituitary	• negative and positive feedback effects on LH/FSH • high levels induce the LH surge • increases TRH and GnRH receptor numbers • increases oxytocin production	• enhances the function of serotonin receptors in brain
Ovary	• is essential for ovum maturation • induces the proliferation of the granulosa cells • induces expression of LH receptors in granulosa cells	• Inhibits follicular development
Vagina	• causes proliferation and cornification of the mucosa	• Inhibits estrogen induced cornification
Oviducts	• causes growth and development in preparation for gamete transport	• maintains secretions
Mammary Glands	• causes growth and development of ducts as well as deposition of fat • increases oxytocin receptors	• is necessary for lobular-alveolar development • decreases prolactin receptors
Skin	• induces sebaceous gland secretion (thinner fluid) • stimulates axillary and pubic hair growth	
Uterus: Cervix	• increases mucus secretion	• increases mucus consistency
Myometrium	• synthesizes contractile proteins of smooth muscle cells • increases membrane excitability (increased sensitivity to oxytocin) • increases blood flow	• causes anti-estrogen effects: decreased sensitivity to oxytocin and decreased estrogen receptor number
Endometrium	• increases prostaglandin synthesis at term, increases oxytocin receptors at term, increases the number of estrogen receptors in the decidua • increases progesterone receptor numbers	• stimulates growth and development in preparation for implantation. Thicker lining, activates glands. • (decrease estrogen receptor number?)
Liver	• causes hepatic angiotensinogen production • causes hepatic production of thyroid-binding globulin	• reduces gallbladder activity
Blood	• decreases plasma cholesterol formation	
General Body	• causes water and sodium retention, weight gain, and female type fat distribution • maintains bone mineralization • tends to increase inflammation	• causes thermogenic action (increase in basal metabolic rate) • is antagonistic to estrogen effects • anti-inflammatory, anti-spasmodic

Estrogen is the name applied to a group of related steroids: estradiol, estriol, estrone and their metabolites. Figure 7 gives the structures of the estradiol, estriol, and estrone as well as their synthetic pathways.

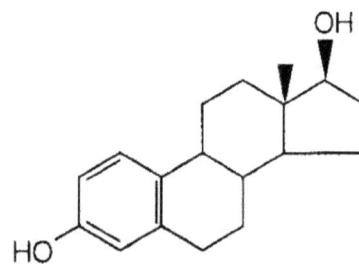
Estradiol

17-beta estradiol is the predominant estrogen released by the ovary. It is metabolized to a mixture of estriol and estrones. The estrones include 4 and 16 alpha-hydroxyestrone which are associated with increased risk of cancer and 2-hydroxyestrone which is considered protective. One of the ways we can work to balance female reproductive hormones is by using herbs and foods that shift metabolic pathways to decrease the harmful estrogen forms.

Progesterone is the major progestogen in the body, but its effects extend far beyond its role in maintaining pregnancy. Of particular interest, progesterone is known to reduce cravings for addictive substances (nicotine, cocaine) and also reduce the subjective reward for using drugs. And, while estrogen is somewhat inflammatory in action, progesterone helps to cool out the body. It balances the effects of estrogen and can act independently as an anti-inflammatory agent.

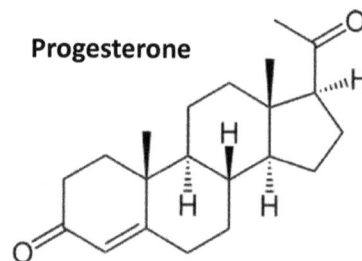
Progesterone

BALANCING THE MENSTRUAL CYCLE

Western Constitutional Model

It is common in many self-help books on women's health to find lists of symptoms and the treatments that assist in alleviating them. For instance, you may find menstrual cramps listed as a problem and cramp bark or essential fatty acids listed as a solution. For each of your issues you can find a specific solution. Using a single herb to deal with an issue is called simpling. It follows an allopathic model. In allopathic medicine, diseases and symptoms are treated with a drug or herb that will counter the effect of the symptom.

This treatise deviates slightly from that approach by challenging the reader to identify what is a happening on a deeper level. While ultimately the treatment may be similar, the understanding of what is creating the imbalance can allow for more creative, comprehensive, and effective change. Women with menstrual cramps generally fall into two of three constitutional patterns which will be presented in the next section.

It is not possible, due to space and time limitations, to explain the entire western constitutional model. However, it is possible to give the reader a taste of how a deep understanding of the body's physiology can open up creative solutions to issues that may arise. For instance, understanding that a menstrual cramp is simply a smooth muscle cramp allows one to realize that any remedy for smooth muscle cramps, such as adequate calcium/magnesium, kava-kava, or catnip, may all work well. In addition, since a cramp or muscle spasm represents hyperactivity of the muscle, calming the body's reactivity in general by use of relaxation methods or supportive nutrition is also valuable. Further, sometimes stimulating the tissue short term may restore balance to the cramping muscle. In this case, a good 'ole fashion orgasm may give immediate relief.

I challenge the reader to begin to see the connections between all aspects of their body health.

Many people have constitutions that run "hot", while others have constitutions that run "cold". Some people dry out and others are moist. Some people run slow, while others run fast. Picking the appropriate remedy or most effective solution requires a deep understanding of how your individual body operates.

Deficient Estrogen Pattern

Follicle development is slow or deficient. This results in low estrogen production which in turn results in reduced follicle development. It is a vicious cycle. Estrogen is needed for follicle development and follicle development is needed for estrogen production. Cycles are longer – typically with longer follicular phase. But since poor follicle development leads to poor CL there may be regular length cycles with long follicular phase and short luteal phase. Luteal phase problems may arise since estrogen, while deficient, may be "louder" than deficient progesterone. Infertility may be present. Other attributes may include light menstrual flow (but lengthy), PMS, absence of breast tenderness and water weight gain, not a lot of cramping.

Follicular development is reduced when estrogen production is low, prolactin is high, FSH production is low and/or stress is high. Stress probably affects developing follicles by a number of mechanisms, but one way is by elevating prolactin. So if the goal is to get better follicular development then the natural approach would be to reduce stress, boost estrogen and/or decrease prolactin. Due to the overlapping nature of follicular development it may take several cycles before full benefit is realized.

Deficient Oxytocin

Deficient estrogen is often accompanied by deficient oxytocin action. Estrogen is responsible for stimulating oxytocin production as well as creating receptors for the oxytocin hormone. Deficient oxytocin is characterized by boring or mellow orgasms, since the pleasurable "punch" of an orgasm is due to contraction that is mediated by oxytocin. Other signs of low oxytocin include lack of genital/nipple sensitivity and infertility. If you feel a sharp pain at ovulation, breast/nipple tenderness, and strong menstrual cramps oxytocin levels are high. Adequate oxytocin is also necessary for healthy corpus luteum formation.

Production of oxytocin can also be reduced due to drinking too much alcohol, smoking marijuana, anorexia, heavy stress, depression, elevated cortisol levels, and pituitary dysfunction or tumor.

Shifting the deficient estrogen pattern

Support estrogen (estrogen agonists):

Plants:

> Black cohosh (*Cimicifuga*)
> Tang Kwei (*Angelica*)
> Red Clover (*Trifolium*)
> Alfalfa (*Medicago*)
> Soybeans (*Glycine max*)

See Table one for the effects of estrogen. Here is a summary:

- increases cervical and vaginal mucus
- increases menstrual flow
- increases oxytocin receptors
- increases nipple sensitivity
- builds up more contractile uterine tissue
- affects calcium absorption
- important in development and release of the egg

While estrogen tends to be inflammatory in nature, all the herbal estrogen mimetics also have anti-inflammatory properties.

Mimic Oxytocin:

> Blue Cohosh (*Caulophyllum*)
> Wild Cotton Root (*Gossypium*)

Reduce prolactin:

> Vitex agnus-castus

Increase Progesterone Activity:

> Vitex agnus-castus (increases LH)
> Dioscorea (potentiates progesterone)

Reduce stress:

Lifestyle changes: meditation, relaxation, exercise, life coaching

Herbs: Adaptogens:

> Eleutherococcus
> Ashwagandha (*Withania*)

Nervines: Avena
Skullcap
Vervain
Motherwort (*Leonurus*)
etc.

NOTES:

Estrogen Excess Pattern

Follicular development is robust. Follicular phase may be shortened with overall cycle shorter. Estrogen dominance is characterized by water retention, breast tenderness, weight gain, cramping, heavy flow and moodiness. If the menstrual flow is heavy that indicates high estrogen. If it is also thick, then progesterone is high as well.

The goal here is to reduce estrogen or at least attenuate the undesirable effects of high estrogen.

Shifting the estrogen excess pattern

Use herbs that mimic estrogen:
Black Cohosh, Tang Kwei, Soybeans, Red Clover, Alfalfa

Even though estrogen is high, the same herbs that are used to support estrogen levels are used in some cases. The proposed mechanism of action is that they compete or displace the endogenous estrogen and/or they "overload" the system causing the body to down-regulate receptors for estrogen. So even though there is lots of estrogen around, the "estrogen response" is lower since the tissue is not responding to it.

Increase Progesterone Activity:
"Progesterone shouts loudest". This means that adequate progesterone can balance out elevated estrogen by cancelling out some of the effects of estrogen.

Herbs: Vitex agnus-castus (increases LH)
           Dioscorea (potentiates progesterone)

Change estrogen metabolism:
Food:
Broccoli, Kale, Cabbage or other brassica family vegetables. They contain a compound that shifts estrogen metabolism from the high inflammatory 4 and 16 OH forms to the "good" 2-OH form.

Liver cooling herbs:
Dandelion Root
Burdock
Dandelion leaf (especially with water retention)

Other: Vitamin C, bioflavonoids and exercise support more efficient metabolism of estrogen

Reduce cramping
Evening Primrose Oil, Borage Oil or other EFA all during the month to prevent. Also helps with moodiness.

Acutely use smooth muscle relaxants. Here they are in order of strength
Catnip, fennel
Dioscorea (wild yam), Kava Kava
Cramp bark (Viburnum opulus),
Garrya (Silk Tassel)
*datura, belladona (atropine) * Not recommended for menstrual cramps. These are poisonous.

Food: Some people find reduction in grains reduces inflammatory tone of body. In addition, the fatty acids in meat and dairy contribute to uterine cramping. Shifting the diet to be more plant based can help eliminate cramping and other forms of inflammation.

NOTES:

<u>Deficient Progesterone (estrogen unopposed)</u>

In this pattern many of the characteristics of the estrogen excess pattern are observed in addition to luteal phase defects. Estrogen production is robust and some progesterone is produced but the CL isn't producing enough progesterone to counteract the inflammatory nature of estrogen. Or the CL drops production before the menses begin resulting in what is commonly referred to as PMS.

All the herbs and strategies listed for estrogen excess are applicable. The major addition is the use of ***Vitex-agnus castus*** which has been validated by sufficient research for the treatment of the deficient progesterone pattern. The other herb is **wild yam** which has not been researched sufficiently yet, but appears to interact in the body to potentiate the actions of progesterone.

Increase Progesterone Activity:

Vitex agnus-castus (increases LH)
Dioscorea (potentiates progesterone)

NOTES:

Birth Control Pills

Two general types of birth control pills are used in the United States. Predominately, women use a combined oral contraceptive that contains both estrogen and progestin. Alternatively, there is a form that contains only progestin and is referred to as the mini pill.

Given what you now know about the control of the menstrual cycle, what would happen if you started adding a whole lot of exogenous (from the outside) estrogen? Starting at the top of the body first, GnRH would be suppressed, which would then lead to a reduction in LH and FSH. This in turn would result in a reduction in the development of follicles. However, since there is a whole lot of estrogen circulating the uterine lining would develop just fine. Ideally, ovulation does not occur because the follicles cannot develop well without FSH. To the body the extra estrogen without FSH means you are pregnant.

No ovulation, means no corpus luteum, and no endogenous (from the inside) production of progesterone. Instead, the pill creates an artificial luteal phase by providing synthetic progesterone. When the progesterone is discontinued, the uterine lining is shed and menses occur.

While some women find that birth control regulates and reduces unpleasant menstrual related issues, others may find that the pill gives them side effects, increases previous complaints or simply doesn't relieve issues like cramping, headaches, etc. In addition, women who take oral contraceptives have a small increased risk for cardiovascular diseases like blood clots, heart attacks, and stroke.[3] The risk of endometrial and ovarian cancers is reduced with the use of birth control pills, while the risk of breast, liver, and cervical cancers is increased.[4]

Now consider the fact that normal follicular development takes a year to complete. How long will it take to return to a balanced cycle after suppressing FSH for any length of time? This can vary, but some women find their cycles are erratic for a year. Using a combination of a estrogen mimetic and a herb like Vitex (which helps restore normal FSH and LH) may coordinate cycles faster.

THE MENOPAUSAL TRANSITION

Characteristics of Perimenopause, Menopause and Postmenopause

As women age, the number of viable follicles that begin developing decreases. This results in a reduced production of estrogen. This can cause a number of problems starting in the perimenopause. Low estrogen production may lead to "wimpy" follicle development followed by a "wimpy" corpus luteum. An underdeveloped corpus luteum will lead to low levels of progesterone and increased symptoms of PMS as well as shorter cycles. This type of pattern responds well to the Vitex agnus-castus which is commonly used for all luteal defects and PMS.

In other cases, the estrogen may never get high enough to induce ovulation or may take longer to do so. The result is longer cycles. No ovulation means no corpus luteum and no progesterone. No clear signal from the ovary to the uterus can lead to break through bleeding during the cycle. In addition, if a period is missed or the cycle lengthened, when the menses actually occur, extremely heavy bleeding may result. These sorts of menstrual irregularities are addressed in the previous chapter.

The changing hormonal climate leads many women to experience some of the following:
- Hot flashes: The experience of being over heated. These can range from an occasional flush to intense heat with full body sweating occurring twelve or more times a day.

- Neurovegetative complaints: Moodiness, anxiety, depression, sleep disturbances.

- Erratic menstrual cycles, eventually ceasing. (Menopause is defined as the absence of menstrual bleeding for one year.)

- Change in estrogen influenced diseases such as fibroids, migraines, and arthritis.

41

Finally, the production of estrogen and progesterone by the ovary ceases. Some estrogen is still produced by the body from peripheral metabolism (in fat, liver, kidneys) of adrenal androstenedione. Since estrogen inhibits the production of GnRH and LH, the hypothalamus responds initially to the decreased levels of estrogen by producing more GnRH. Given the proximity of where the GnRH is produced and the location of the thermoregulatory center in the brain it seems reasonable that the high levels of GnRH are interacting with the temperature center causing a temporary dysregulation.

A hot flash occurs after a surge of GnRH when the thermoregulatory center momentarily senses that body temperature has risen and sends commands to the body to cool off. The result is redirection of blood to the surface (the feeling of heat and flushing) and activation of other cooling mechanisms such as sweating. While some women welcome hot flashes, most women find them disruptive. The hot flash is experienced by 95% of women that undergo surgical menopause (removal of ovaries) and 75% of women during natural menopause.[5]

If high levels of GnRH are involved in the etiology of hot flashes then it would be expected that administration of estrogen and estrogen agonists would reduce the frequency of hot flashes due to their negative feedback action which serves to reduce GnRH. Therefore it isn't surprising that estrogen is extremely effective in reducing hot flashes clinically and in animal models.[6] Similarly the herbs that mimic estrogen, like black cohosh, are also extremely effective in reducing hot flashes.[7,8,9,10] In addition, herbs that influence neural pathways and/or have a "cooling" effect on the body can also effectively relieve hot flashes.

Table 1 (page 31), which lists the actions of estrogen and progesterone, can be referred to for clues on what to expect when the ovary stops producing these hormones. In addition to the cessation of menses and hot flashes, vaginal tissue can become dry, sexual desire can decrease, and bones can thin.

The Solution

Mainstream medicine offers Hormone Replacement Therapy (HRT) for the alleviation of complaints that accompany the climacteric. This solution is not without problems, which includes the fact that it merely delays the issue; HRT is only recommended short term. When women terminate HRT symptoms may resume at full strength, since the treatment was only suppressive.

In the next section, HRT is explained and then the alternatives to HRT are presented. The advantage of the alternatives is that they work with the body to restore balance. In general, they are gentler and safer to use long term than pharmaceuticals. In addition, the alternative therapies are designed to allow a woman's body to complete the transition from the higher levels of hormones to reduced levels without unpleasant effects.

Hormone Replacement Therapy (HRT)

There are three general types of commonly prescribed HRT

- estrogen only HRT
- combined HRT - estrogen every day with progesterone and progestin added for 10-14 days each month
- continuous combined HRT - estrogen and progestin every day continuously

Some Oral Estrogen Products

Premarin (**PRE**gnant **MAR**es' ur**IN**e) conjugated horse estrogens - This is considered "natural" estrogen. It is made from the urine of pregnant horses, which means that the pregnant mares are fitted with a urine collection device and held in small stalls for six months of the year. Activists are working to eliminate this form of animal cruelty. (For more info: www.premarin.org)

Cenestin synthetic conjugated estrogens

Estratab esterified estrogens

Menest esterified estrogens

Ortho-Est estropipate (piperazine estrone sulfate)

Ogen estropipate (piperazine estrone sulfate)

Estrace micronized 17-betaestradiol

Estinyl ethinyl estradiol

Some Oral Progestin Products (Progestin is a synthetic form of progesterone.)

Cycrin medroxyprogesterone acetate

Provera medroxyprogesterone acetate

Aygestin norethindrone acetate

Norlutate norethindrone acetate

Prometrium progesterone USP (in peanut oil) - this is "natural" progesterone that is synthesized from yams in the laboratory.

Estrogen-plus-progestin pills

Premphase conjugated horse estrogens and medroxyprogesterone acetate

Prempro conjugated horse estrogens and medroxyprogesterone acetate

Femhrt ethinyl estradiol and norethindrone acetate

Activella 17-beta-estradiol and norethindrone acetate

Ortho-Prefest 17-beta-estradiol and norgestimate

Also available

Estrogen in vaginal creams, skin creams, patches and vaginal inserts. Progesterone in vaginal gel. Combined estrogen and progesterone skin patch.

Dr. Lois Johnson is an herbalist and a physician that I studied with and made medicine for. She uses predominantly herbs in her practice. While she avoids synthetic hormones including Premarin, she will use natural hormones when the person is at risk for severe osteoporosis and/or heart disease.

Dr. Johnson recommends that all HRT be done using creams or patches since all hormones are "irritating to the liver" and the transdermal route bypasses the liver. The mildest form of HRT uses natural progesterone cream. This is enough to help some, but not all women. Natural progesterone is available over-the-counter at many health food stores. If you desire to try a estrogen cream, she recommends estriol as a first choice since it is a fairly weak estrogen and has protective effects against breast cancer. In addition, it is great to use for vaginal atrophy. Very small doses are effective when applied topically.

Bezwecken sells both estrogen creams and combination creams to health care practitioners: http://www.bezwecken.com/products.php. You can also order them through my Natural Partners online store: http://www.npscript.com/elderberrycenter You will need the following access code to create an account:

Since it is important to be informed about proper use and risks of using these creams, please contact me to get the access code. DorenaRode@gmail.com. If you have taken the class with me, the code will be in filled in above.

Why you want to avoid medical HRT

The following is reprinted (with minor edits) from *"Facts About Menopausal Hormone Therapy"*[11]

The Women's Health Initiative

In 1991, the National Heart, Lung, and Blood Institute (NHLBI) and other units of the National Institutes of Health (NIH) launched the Women's Health Initiative (WHI), one of the largest studies of its kind ever undertaken in the United States. It consists of a set of clinical trials, an observational study, and a community prevention study, which altogether involve more than

161,000 healthy postmenopausal women.

The menopausal hormone therapy clinical trial had two parts. The first involved 16,608 postmenopausal women with a uterus who took either estrogen plus- progestin therapy or a placebo. (The added progestin protects women against uterine cancer.) The second involved 10,739 women who had had a hysterectomy and took estrogen alone or a placebo. (A placebo is a substance that looks like the real drug but has no biologic effect.) The estrogen-plus-progestin trial used 0.625 milligrams of conjugated equine estrogens taken daily plus 2.5 milligrams of dedroxyprogesterone acetate (PremproTM) taken daily. The estrogen-alone trial used 0.625 milligrams of conjugated equine estrogens (PremarinTM) taken daily. Prempro and Premarin were chosen for two key reasons: They contain the most commonly prescribed forms of estrogen-alone and combined therapies in the United States, and, in several observational studies, these drugs appeared to benefit women's health. Both hormone studies were to have continued until 2005, but were stopped early. The estrogen plus-progestin study was halted in July 2002, and the estrogen-alone study at the end of February 2004.

Effects on Disease and Death
Briefly, the combination therapy study was stopped because of an increased risk of breast cancer and because, overall, risks from use of the hormones outnumbered the benefits. "Outnumbered" means that more women had adverse effects from the therapy than benefited from it. For breast cancer, the risk was greatest among women who had used estrogen plus progestin before entering the study, indicating that the therapy may have a cumulative effect. The combination therapy also increased the risk for heart attack, stroke, and blood clots. For heart attack, the risk was particularly high in the first year of hormone use and continued for several years thereafter. There was an overall increased risk from the hormone therapy over the 5.6 years of the trial. The risk for blood clots was greatest during the first 2 years of hormone use—four times higher than that of placebo users. By the end of the study, the risk for blood clots had decreased to two times greater—or 18 more women with blood clots each year for every 10,000 women. Estrogen plus progestin also reduced the risk for hip and other fractures, and colorectal cancer. The reduction in colorectal cancer risk appeared after 3 years of hormone use and became more marked thereafter. However, the number of cases of colorectal cancer was relatively small, and more research is needed to confirm the finding.

The estrogen-alone study was stopped after almost 7 years because the hormone therapy increased the risk of stroke and did not reduce the risk of coronary heart disease. It also increased the risk for venous thrombosis (blood clots deep in a vein, usually in the leg). There also was a trend towards increased risk for pulmonary embolism (blood clots in the lungs), but it was not statistically significant. The therapy had no significant effect on the risk of heart disease or colorectal cancer. Its effect on breast cancer was uncertain. Although the risk for breast cancer for those on estrogen alone appeared to be lower, this finding was not statistically significant. Estrogen alone reduced the risk for hip and other fractures. The reduction began early in the study and persisted throughout the follow up period. Neither estrogen plus progestin nor estrogen alone affected the

Summary of WHI Study Findings

The percentages given below describe what would happen to a whole population—not to an individual woman. For example, breast cancer risk for the women in the WHI study taking estrogen plus progestin increased less than a tenth of 1 percent each year. But if you apply that increased risk to a large group of women over several years, the number of women affected becomes an important public health concern. About 6 million American women take estrogen-plus-progestin therapy. That would translate into nearly 6,000 more breast cancer cases every year, and, if all of the women who took the therapy for 5 years, that could result in 30,000 more breast cancer cases. Further, know that percentages aren't fate. Whether expressing risks or benefits, they do not mean you will develop a disease. Many factors affect that likelihood, including your lifestyle and other environmental factors, heredity, and your personal medical history.

Estrogen Plus Progestin Study

Combined hormone replacement therapy for women with a uterus. These are the results at 5.2 years follow up. For every 10,000 women each year, estrogen plus progestin (combination therapy) use compared with a placebo on average resulted in:

- 26% increased risk for breast cancer
- 41% increased risk for stroke
- 29% increased risk for heart attack
- Twice the risk for blood clots in legs, lungs
- 37% less risk for colorectal cancer
- 37% less risk for hip fractures

Estrogen Alone Study

Hormone replacement therapy for women without uterus (post-hysterectomy). Women in the estrogen-alone study began the trial with a higher risk for cardiovascular disease than those in the estrogen-plus-progestin study. They were more likely to have such heart disease risk factors as high blood pressure, high blood cholesterol, diabetes, and obesity. At 6.8 years follow-up. For every 10,000 women each year, estrogen-alone use compared with a placebo on average resulted in:

- 39% increase risk of stroke
- 47% increased risk of venous thrombosis (blood clot, usually deep vein in legs)
- 39% fewer hip fractures
- No differences in risk for coronary heart disease (trend to increased risk in first two years of estrogen therapy, but decreased risk overall), colorectal cancer, breast cancer (trend to decrease risk).

HRT vs. Birth Control Pills

Very-low-dose birth control pills (LoEstrin 1/20, Alesse) typically have 20 micrograms of estrogen, compared with 30 to 50 micrograms of estrogen in regular birth control pills. HRT, as used in the studies above, delivered 625 micrograms of estrogen a day. However, the synthetic estrogens used in birth control pills are about 50 to 75 times as potent in the body as natural horse estrogens, hence it is estimated that birth control delivers two to four times as much estrogen action to the body as HRT.[12]

Alternative Medicine Approach

The hallmark complaint of the post-menopause period is hot flashes. The overall alternative medicine strategy for reducing or eliminating hot flashes is "cooling" the woman down. There a number of ways to do this. One method may be enough, or many may need to be combined.

1) Reduce Stress

Meditation, relaxation, life coaching, moderate exercise
Adaptogenic herbs:
Siberian Ginseng
Ashwagandha
Schizandra

Nervines:
Hops (insomnia with flushing)
Motherwort (heart palpitations)
Skullcap (general stress and anxiety)
Lavender
Avena
Valerian
Passion flower
etc.

2) Cooling Therapy
Avoid hot foods (curries, peppers, other spicy foods)
Increase cool foods (cucumber, watermelon, cabbage, parsley, raw vegetables)
Avoid sugar, caffeine, fatty foods, alcohol
Chickweed herb
Cool Stuff for Hot Women Tea (Dr. Lois Johnson): Hibiscus (2 parts), Schizandra berries (4 parts), Lemon Balm (1 part), Linden (1 part), Sage (1 part)

3) Foods and herbs that mimic estrogen or estrogen effects
Black cohosh
Tang Kwei
soy beans (isoflavones)
red clover
pomegranates
vitamin C
hesperidin

4) Herbs with specific actions that appear to be helpful
Lobelia
Anemone
Licorice

5) Supplements

Soy Beans
Soy isoflavones are thought to be selective estrogen receptor modulators (SERMs) and as such may act to reduce hot flashes while being safe in terms of breast and uterine cancer risks. However overall research suggests that soy isoflavones are not effective in reducing menopausal symptoms.[13] In addition, there is no conclusive evidence that they can improve bone mineralization either or cognition.[13] However, they may still exert a protective effect on breast and uterine tissue, perhaps competing for receptors with endogenous (and uterine and breast cancer promoting) estrogens.[13]

However, there is good evidence that 25grams of soybean protein consumed each day will reduce overall cholesterol and improve the LDL to HDL balance by increasing HDL and decreasing LDL.[13] Further 100 grams of tofu with 1 tablespoon flax seed has been shown to reduce hot flashes and reduce vaginal dryness.[14]

Promensil, a standardized extract of red clover

Hot flashes: Three studies showed no effect, one study showed decreased hot flashes with 30 mg Promensil per day.[13] Bone Density: Two studies suggest 56 to 85mg/day isoflavones from red clover will increase bone density or at least slow the loss.[13] Effects on lipids: Three studies with no effect and one study with increased HDL. [13]

Vitamin E and Evening Primrose (gamolenic acid)

The scientific literature overall suggests these are not effective for reducing hot flashes, but still are beneficial for overall health, especially cardiovascular health. However, clinical experience suggests that Vitamin E 100 to 500 mg IU does reduce hot flash severity.

Vitamin C, Bioflavonoids, Hesperidin, Rutin

Vitamin C and related bioflavonoids are respected for their important role in collagen formation. Collagen is an important structural protein found in bones and the skin.

In addition, these compounds have a relationship to estrogen that is not well understood. High estrogen states typically lead to lower levels of vitamin C and in some animals vitamin C either acts like estrogen or potentiates estrogenic effects (can lead to abortion). Despite the lack of clear understanding on mechanism of action, there is some evidence that 200mg vitamin C plus 200mg bioflavonoids six times a day relieved hot flashes in 88% of cases. Compared to 72% taking estrogen and 22% taking calcium carbonate.[15]

6) Lifestyle

Keep stress to a minimum, get regular exercise. The most important thing you can do to maintain **healthy bones** is weight bearing exercise such as walking, stair-climbing, dancing, strength training or similar activities. If you are sedentary start with 10 minutes a day three times a week. Eventually work up to 30-60 minutes 3-5 days a week. Some women find that regular aerobic exercise can decrease hot flashes.

7) Food

Consume an overall healthy diet high in fruits and vegetables (about 1.5 pounds a day). Avoid processed food, carbonated beverages, empty calories. Sugar, caffeine, fatty foods, and alcohol tend to make hot flashes worse.

BONE HEALTH

Many people wrongly assume that adequate calcium intake ensures strong bones. Once you understand how bones grow you see the insanity in this simple assumption. This chapter will explain calcium homeostasis, bone remodeling and how to maintain healthy bones.

Calcium is an important chemical messenger in the body and is essential for nerve firing and muscle contractions. The bone serves as a storage area for this important nutrient. Absorption is regulated by vitamin D and ultimately by the body's demand for calcium. The best way to get more calcium absorbed is to create a demand for it by exercising.

Understanding Calcium Balance

Calcium is a regulated essential parameter in the body. Blood levels are held constant (between 9 to 11 mg per deciliter.) Regulation is via negative feedback mechanisms, which means if we have too much calcium in the blood, hormones act to reduce the calcium by excreting it in the urine, slowing absorption from the gut, and stopping the bone from releasing it. In contrast, if blood levels drop, we will retain it at the kidney, absorb more from our guts and break bones down to get more into the blood.

Why do we regulate calcium?
Calcium is important for:
- muscle contractions
- nerve conduction
- signaling the release of hormones and neurotransmitters from a cell
- communication within a cell about what to do in response to external stimulus
- blood clotting; it is a cofactor in the clotting cascade

While 99% of calcium in the body is in the teeth and bones (1.2 to 1.4 kg), only free calcium is biologically active. Most of the calcium not stored in the bones is found within the cells; there is less than 1.5 grams circulating in the blood.

We must keep calcium levels in the blood constant because the ability for the calcium within the cell to perform its function is dependent on the difference between levels inside and outside of the cell (the calcium gradient). Intracellular concentrations of calcium are low. Extracellular concentrations are high. If calcium levels drop in the plasma/interstitial fluid this disrupts the calcium gradient which increases excitability of nerves and muscles. The short story is we end up twitching and we spasming when calcium levels in the blood drop.

Calcium supplementation

I prefer to supplement a balanced ratio of calcium and magnesium. Others advocate more magnesium to calcium, others more calcium to magnesium. Use your intuition or alternate and see if you notice any difference. There simply isn't enough research to give a hard and fast rule here. I use one part calcium to one part magnesium. Despite marketing claims, calcium carbonate is just as easily absorbed as calcium citrate (slight difference that is not clinically significant).

Hypercalcemia

High blood calcium: plasma levels greater than 11mg/dl

High levels of calcium in the blood stimulate the c-cells (also known as parafollicular cells) located in the thyroid gland to release calcitonin. **Calcitonin** is a hormone that acts at the kidney and the bone to reduce the calcium in the blood. *(There is some controversy regarding the significance of calcitonin action at physiological levels.)*

• At the kidney calcitonin acts to increase the urinary excretion of both calcium and phosphate.

• At the bone calcitonin reduces calcium release by slowing bone resorption (the breakdown of bones) by inhibiting the osteoclast cells. See Figure 10.

Figure 10: The action of calcitonin on the bone. (hypercalcemia)

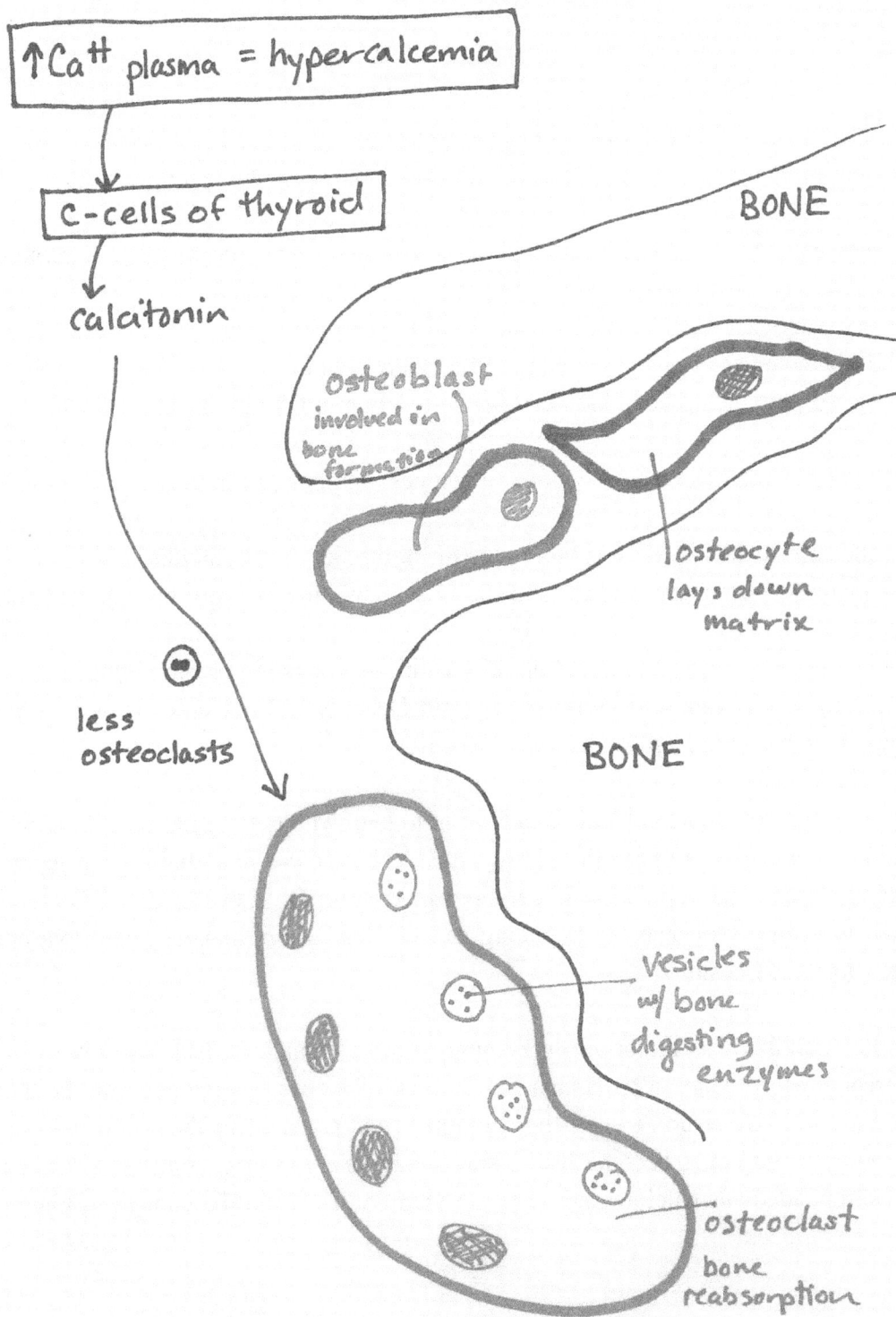

↑Ca⁺⁺ plasma = hypercalcemia

C-cells of thyroid

calcitonin

less osteoclasts

BONE

osteoblast involved in bone formation

osteocyte lays down matrix

BONE

vesicles w/ bone digesting enzymes

osteoclast bone reabsorption

Hypocalcemia

Low blood calcium: plasma levels less than 9mg/dl

See figure 11.

Low levels of calcium in the blood stimulate the parathyroid to release parathyroid hormone (PTH). PTH is a hormone that acts at the kidney and bones to increase the level of calcium in the blood.

- PTH increases calcium reabsorption and phosphate excretion in the distal and proximal tubules of the kidney respectively.
- PTH increases osteoclast activity. This results in increased bone resorption and release of calcium phosphate and calcium carbonate into the blood stream.
- PTH activates the enzyme in the kidney that converts Vitamin D3 into its active form.

Vitamin D3 is a hormone that acts at the kidney, intestines, and bone to increase calcium levels in the blood.

- Vitamin D3 increases calcium reabsorption in the distal tubule. (Less calcium in urine.)
- Vitamin D3 increases osteoclast activity and the release of calcium from the bones. (Bones broken down.)
- Vitamin D3 increases a calcium transport protein (calbindin) in the intestinal lining, allowing for greater absorption of calcium. With no vitamin D3 only 20% of calcium is absorbed. With vitamin D3, 80% of calcium is absorbed. (See figure 11.)

The bottom line is that eating more calcium is not going to help with getting more calcium in the bones. Vitamin D3 is what is regulating how much calcium we absorb. Recent research indicates that close to half the population is deficient in vitamin D. Low levels of vitamin D have been linked to a variety of diseases including cancer, depression, diabetes, cardiovascular disease, hypertension, and obesity.

Notice that while Vitamin D3 is important in helping us absorb calcium, it is also involved in activating the breakdown of bone! This is because the body if focused on maintaining the blood calcium levels constant. If we don't keep the calcium levels constant in the blood we die in minutes/hours, while if the bones become brittle and break we may suffer, but we will not die immediately. Getting adequate calcium and adequate vitamin D will not be enough to maintain bone health.

Figure 11: The action of PTH & Vitamin D3 on maintaining optimal blood calcium levels.

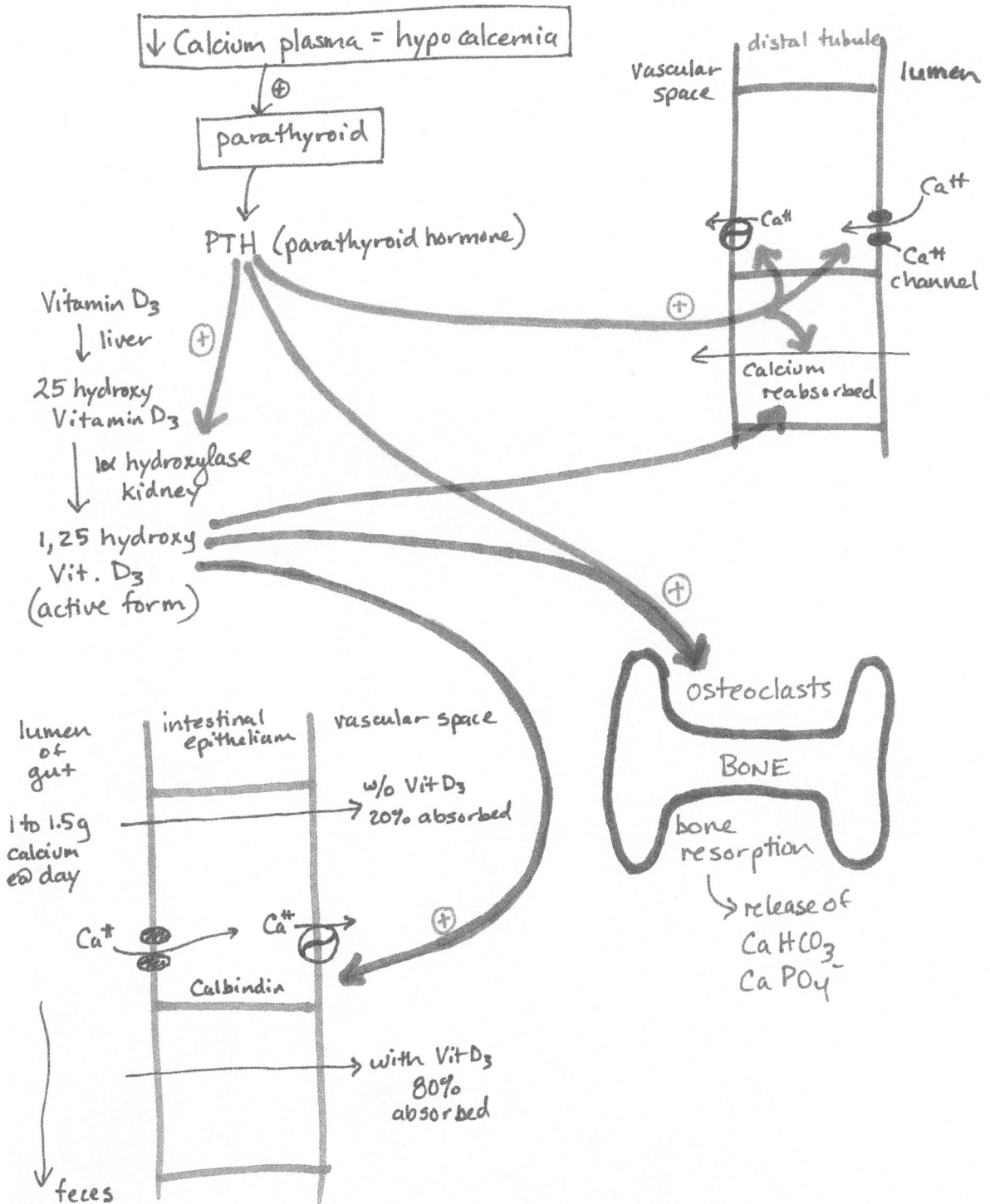

↓ Calcium plasma = hypo calcemia

⊕

parathyroid

PTH (parathyroid hormone)

Vitamin D₃
↓ liver   ⊕

25 hydroxy
Vitamin D₃

↓ 1α hydroxylase
kidney

1,25 hydroxy
Vit. D₃
(active form)

distal tubule

vascular space   lumen

Ca⁺⁺
Ca⁺⁺

Ca⁺⁺
channel

⊕

Calcium reabsorbed

⊕

osteoclasts

BONE

bone resorption
↳ release of
Ca HCO₃
Ca PO₄⁻

lumen of gut

intestinal epithelium   vascular space

w/o Vit D₃
20% absorbed

1 to 1.5g calcium e@ day

Ca⁺   Ca⁺⁺   ⊕
Calbindin

with Vit D₃
80% absorbed

↓ feces

Figure 12: Bone Remodeling

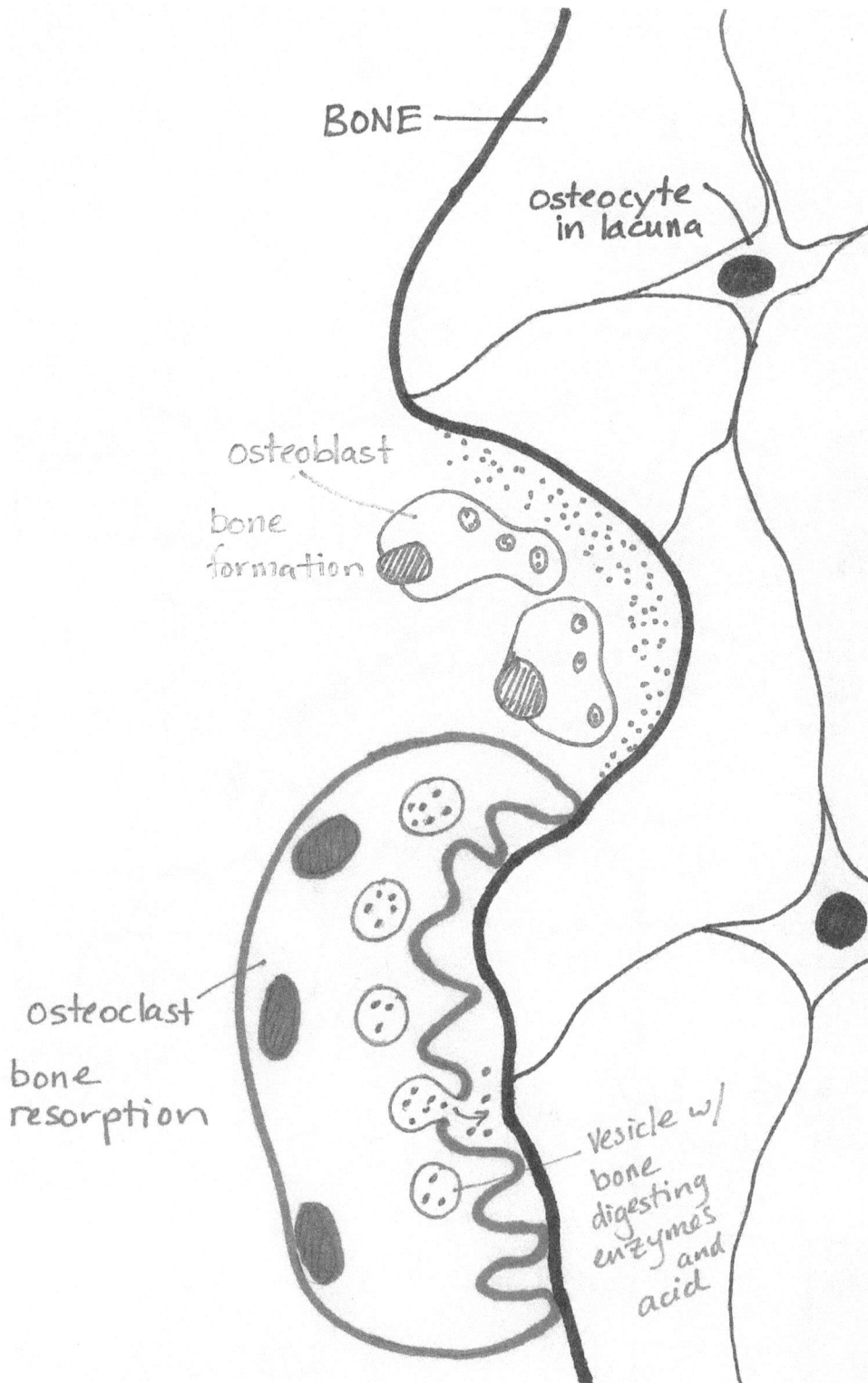

BONE

osteocyte in lacuna

osteoblast

bone formation

osteoclast

bone resorption

Vesicle w/ bone digesting enzymes and acid

Bone Remodeling

Another misconception is that bones are a static, solid thing. In truth they are a dynamic, constantly changing tissue. Actually, about 10% of the skeleton is completely remodeled every year. The rate of turnover depends on the bone and the amount of physical stress it encounters.

The bone in the skeleton can be divided into two types. Compact or **cortical bone** makes up about 80% of the skeleton. It is the dense, solid bone that surrounds a marrow cavity, like the shaft of the leg bone. This type of bone turns over at rate of about 3% each year. The other 20% of the skeleton is made up of spongy or **trabecular bone**. It looks more like a solidified sponge when sliced open. Trabecular bone makes up the majority of the ends of long bones and much of the bones in the vertebral column. This type of bone encounters more stress and turns over at a rate of 25% a year.

Bone remodeling is accomplished by the activity of two cells (See Figure 12). The **osteoclasts** are large macrophage like cells that release enzymes and acids that break down the bone and release the calcium and minerals. When osteoclasts break down bone it is called bone resorption. The **osteoblasts** are smaller cells that work in groups to lay down a collagen rich matrix that they subsequently mineralize with a calcium-phosphate-hydroxide salt (hydroxyapatite). This process is called bone formation.

Estrogen, testosterone, thyroid hormones, and growth hormone all stimulate osteoblasts to create more bone. Estrogen and calcitonin inhibit the activity of osteoclasts.

How to Build Bone

1) Weight bearing exercise.
Walk! Bicycling does not have the same protective effects as walking and running. Tai chi and chi gung have the added benefit of specifically increasing bone density. There is a reason Tai chi is considered an essential component of longevity practices. Bone responds to physical stress by getting stronger. It is a simple as that.

2) Herbs and nutrients that mimic or modulate estrogen, thyroid and growth hormone.

Estrogen modulators: Black cohosh   Tang Kwei   red clover
                       soy beans (isoflavones)   pomegranates   vitamin C
                       hesperidin

3) Adequate protein, calcium, minerals, and vitamin D3

4) Decrease stress.

Corticosteroids that are released during stress result in skin thinning and weaken bones.

5) Slow resorption by alkalizing body.

 Bone loss can occur when the body pH is acidic, since bone is broken down to release phosphate and other buffers. This may not be significant, but worthy of consideration. There is also some evidence that a high protein diet may increase bone turnover.[16] Again, this clinical significance of this is questionable.   It is also possible that an alkaline diet may support bone health by increasing growth hormone.[17]

6) Avoid Caffeine and Colas.

The caffeine found in about four cups of coffee (330 mg/day) has been associated with a greater risk of bone fractures.[18] In addition, there is also an association between cola/soda consumption and decrease in bone density.[19]   Further, phosphorus (a common ingredient in colas) also increases bone resorption and decreases the markers for bone formation.

Bone Resorption Visualization

Get comfortable, sit up, lie down, any position that feels right.

Feel yourself relaxing fully. Feel yourself heavy. Feel your body fully. Feel the places where your body connects with the earth, the ground, or other solid objects. Feel the pressure. Relax. Relax, let the solid objects support you. Feel your connection to the earth. (Big breaths.)

Now, from the heaven, begins a shower of golden energy. Sparkling star dust showers down upon you. Your aura, your person, your being is cleansed by this golden energy shower. Everything and everyone is washed clean from your space. You are renewed. You are free. Just you and your connection to the divine remains.

You feel your connection. You feel connected to the earth; You are at peace with yourself. Feel yourself. The movement of your breath, the pulse of the river of life within you, you feel deep into the core of your being, your awareness moves everywhere within you. You feel deep into your bones. Bring your awareness to the center of your thigh bones - the femurs. Feel them solid within you. Feel how solid you are. Solid like the earth.

Move to the central space within the bones. The femur has a hollow core surrounded by compact bone. Bring your focus into that hollow space. You can imagine yourself very small standing in that space. The cavity is filled with a yellow bone marrow. This marrow is made up of many cells filled with fat. The fat cells are bathed in interstitial fluid. This is the fluid of life that bathes all the cells in the body. It is fresh and vibrant. Blood vessels run the length of the space.

Imagine yourself following a blood vessel down your leg inside the bone towards the end of the femur at the knee. You enter an area of spongy bone. It is like a great room with honeycomb scaffolding. Stay within this spongy bone area. You are within the mineral/protein structure of the bones. See the chambers and spaces. The spaces are filled with bone marrow. You see, near the solid bone, two types of cells.

The first cell is small and has a slightly irregular shape. It is an osteoblast cell. These cells are close to the bone. Look closely and you can see they are slowly, gently secreting a liquid protein and mineral solution. They are laying down this gel like substance next to solid bone. Over the next week the minerals will crystallize within the protein matrix and become solid new bone. Osteoblasts form new bone. They do this day in and day out.

The second type of cell is much, much bigger. It is 10 times the size of the osteoblast. It is an osteoclast cell. Now, move your awareness into an osteoclast cell; become an osteoclast. Feel your amoeboid body. You are a bone resorption cell. You are an osteoclast. Look yourself over. You are like a bag of jelly with many small nuclei. Feel your boundaries - your cell membrane. Feel how it moves with the proteins imbedded in it floating around. All parts of you are active and alive.

You are a mobile cell. You move and slide along the bone surface. You touch a neighboring osteoblast cell. You feel this connection through the proteins floating in your cell membrane. These proteins extend through the cell membrane and connect with your internal matrix. Information about the outside world is communicated to your entire being. You respond to this information by initiating enzyme cascades and shifting the flow of messenger proteins. You are infinitely complex and dynamic.

Because you are an osteoclast cell you have a special purpose. You resorb bone. To do this you produce vesicles filled with digestive chemicals. The chemicals are formed in your endoplasmic reticulum, further processed in your Golgi apparatus, and then stored in vesicles within the jelly matrix of your cytosol. Communication from the outside triggers a cascade of events that culminates in the vesicles merging with your cell membrane and releasing the digestive contents onto the bone. The bone melts away and the minerals and proteins of the bone are recycled, reused. Then new bone is formed to replace the old.

Bone remodeling is occurring all the time. Osteoblasts forming bone and osteoclasts resorbing the old bone. Bone is solid and firm and also dynamic and alive. Continuously changing, continuously made new. The process of eating away old bone and laying down new bone is referred to as bone turn-over.

You have experienced a lot and now your time as an osteoclast cell comes to an end. Leave the osteoclast and move your awareness back into your bones. Feel your bones in your legs. This is your grounding. Breath.

As you widen your awareness to the include the room and what lies ahead of you, remember all the answers are within you. Your body is in balance and works well. You have a dynamic connection with the divine. Feel free to get up and resume what you were doing at a pace that suits you.

MATERIA MEDICA

Cross Reference List

The list of herbs is presented in alphabetical order by scientific name. Use this cross reference list to find the Latin name that corresponds with the common name.

Acanthopanax - ELEUTHEROCOCCUS
Ashwagandha - WITHANIA SOMNIFERA
Barberry - BERBERIS
Bearberry - ARCTOSTAPHYLOS
Berberis - MAHONIA
Bethroot - TRILLIUM
Black Cohosh - CIMICIFUGA
Black Haw - VIBURNUM
Blue Cohosh - CAULOPHYLLUM
Bugleweed - LYCOPUS
Burdock - ARCTIUM
California Mugwort - ARTEMISIA VULGARIS
California Snakeroot - ASARUM
Catnip - NEPETA
Chaste Tree Berries - VITEX AGNUS-CASTUS
Cohosh, Black - CIMICIFUGA
Cohosh, Blue - CAULOPHYLLUM
Cotton Root - GOSSYPIUM
Cramp Bark - VIBURNUM
Damiana - TURNERA
Dandelion - TARAXACUM

Dong Quai - ANGELICA SINENSIS
Fennel - FOENICULUM
Feverfew - CHRYSANTHEUM
Ginger - ZINGIBER
Ginger, Wild - ASARUM
Ginseng, Siberian - ELEUTHEROCOCCUS
Ginseng, Indian -WITHANIA SOMNIFERA
Jasmine, Yellow - GELSEMIUM
Kava Kava - PIPER METHYSTICUM
Kinnikinnik - ARCTOSTAPHYLOS
Lappa - ARCTIUM
Macrotys - CIMICIFUGA
Manzanita - ARCTOSTAPHYLOS
Marigold, Common - CALENDULA
Milkweed, Butterfly - ASCLEPIAS TUBEROSA
Monks Pepper - VITEX AGNUS-CASTUS
Motherwort - LEONURUS
Mugwort - ARTEMISIA VULGARIS
Nettles - URTICA
Oats - AVENA
Ocotillo - FOUQUIERIA
Passion Flower - PASSIFLORA
Poke Root - PHYTOLACCA
Quinine Bush - GARRYA
Red Cedar - THUJA
Sage - SALVIA
Sage, White - SALVIA APIANA
Saw Palmetto - SERENOA
Shepherd's Purse - CAPSELLA
Silk Tassel - GARRYA
Skullcap - SCUTELLARIA
Tang Kwei - ANGELICA SINENSIS
Thlaspi - CAPSELLA
Uva Ursi - ARCTOSTAPHYLOS
White Sage - SALVIA APIANA
Wild Ginger - ASARUM
Wild Yam - DIOSCOREA
Witch Hazel - HAMAMELIS

Yellow Cedar - THUJA
Yellow Dock - RUMEX CRISPUS
Yellow Jasmine - GELSEMIUM
Yellow Pond Lily - NUPHAR

Source of this Materia Medica

The information presented in this Materia Medica came predominately from course lectures given by Adam Seller of the Pacific School of Medicine. While I have incorporated my own experiences with the herbs, my experience pales in comparison to Adam's and it seems like a disservice to waste the valuable information he so freely gave. However, since I cannot validate some of the material, I would recommend the reader use the information provided with caution as I may have made errors in transcription or understanding. (Although I did compare my notes with the notes of a student that attended the school during a different time period.)

Despite the limitations of passing on information from another source, I believe this materia medica will contribute to the value of this treatise more than if I simply referred to the herbs in passing and left the reader to figure out more about each herb independently. In addition, the short nature of the course that this book accompanies, prevents me from important details using the plant. This reference serves to complete the classroom material. Also, some of the herbs that I mention and personally use simply cannot be found in the mainstream press, hence the importance of this section.

ANEMONE *Pulsatilla*

If you match the proper nervine with a person the results are immediate and dramatic: 30seconds to 2 minutes. Anemone nervine profile: The person is cold, clammy, pale, dark, nervous, empty, scared, doom and gloom, nightmares (especially of being chased with knives, twisted flesh, dull eyes.)   This herb often suits people dealing with sexual abuse. Sometimes people are wired and active, but with a sense of being contained. When they seem relaxed they are more apt to be low energy than relaxed. Internally tortured.

Properties: Helps recalibrate corticotropic releasing hormone (CRH) and dopamine levels.
- Mild vasodilator.
- Decreases cerebral spinal fluid (CSF) pressure and intraocular pressure. These often increase with onset of migraines.

Preparation: Fresh plant tincture.

Contraindications: Extremely powerful, use in very small doses and with caution. Signs of excess dose: bradycardia; increase in parasympathetic tone (person will become cold and clammy); will make throat burn.

Uses/Dosage: Dosage: *small amounts are very effective*. Seldom require more than 5 drops at a time, though may need every few hours. Often one drop/day divided into 6 doses. Homeopathic 6X is good.
- PMS moodiness with the desire to maim and kill, high estrogen, and intense sugar cravings.
-Anemone has special focus on the gonads. Dopamine excess affects corpus luteum, ovaries, fallopian tubes. Pain in fallopian tubes and uterus almost instantly responds to anemone. Sharp pain with ovulation and uterine pain.
- Not lactating due to stress- often a drop will help.
- Thyroid excess or deficiency developed as response to stress. Works on how the hypothalamus regulates the thyroid, not directly on thyroid.

ANGELICA SINENSIS *Dang Gui, Dong Quai, Tang Kwei.*

This refers to *Angelica sinensis* rhizome that has undergone traditional Chinese processing that may include soaking, steaming, boiling or frying in Chinese wine, rice vinegar, juice or ginger.

Properties: Acts like an estrogen agonist. Liver anabolic.

Preparation: Tincture of cured rhizome 1:5 in 70% alcohol. Decoction tends to be laxative.

Contraindications: Pregnancy or subclinical gonad hyperfunction; aldosterone-induced essential hypertension or any subclinical anabolic excess state.

Uses/Dosage: 250 – 500 mg rhizome (5 - 20 drops tincture) to four times a day
Dong quai has similar indications as Black Cohosh. This is preferred in people that tend towards constipation, since it is more laxative. Flavor is sweet and aromatic compared to *Cimicifuga*.

-Use when mucosa is dry: uterus, labia, cervix, vagina, eyes, throat, gut, skin
-Low estrogen types may find it hard to sleep, low sex drive, dry tissues. Angelica can help these symptoms, though usually not enough alone, need to combine.
-Gets better utilization of oxytocin
-Use with catabolic constitutional type (brittle hair, nails, and blood sugar yo-yos.)

Combinations: Use with *Ceanothus* for ovarian cysts with low estrogen.

ARCTIUM *Burdock*

Properties: Important constitutional remedy for anabolic types. Burdock contains inulin, a soluble fiber fructan, that helps to balance gut flora and promote intestinal health. Cools liver down.
-Mild diuretic, slightly reduces high blood pressure, improves secretion of uric acid
-Reduces LDL's and VLDL's and possibly triglycerides
-Increases fluid excretion by liver, but not bile salts

Preparation: Fresh roots can be eaten or juiced. These can be found in the produce section of the supermarket. Simmer dry root 1/2 hour then bring to boil, then simmer an additional hour.

Uses/Dosage: Use 1/3 to 1 oz dry root per day as a decoction.
- Use when androgens or estrogen/progesterone are high. These hormones can result in water

retention that burdock will correct.

-Very good for eczema, psoriasis, chronic boils, and conditions with elevated IgE. IgE becomes elevated when someone is stressed (elevated adrenalin). Elevated IgE in seen in allergies, eczema, asthma, Crohn's, etc.

Combinations: Combine with licorice for its aldosterone like effect (antidiuretic) if using it with people that run a lot of adrenaline and urinate a lot already.

ARCTOSTAPHYLOS   *Uva Ursi, Manzanita*

Properties: Astringent, tightens protein collagen structures anywhere, internal or external. Mild vasoconstrictor. Sometimes called toxic, but the toxic compounds (hydroxyquinolines) are formed in the kidney and directly excreted, so it is not important. The compounds are toxic to urinary tract infection bacteria as well as the host. Effective with *E. Coli*, works if urine is acidic or alkaline. Berries are very high in vitamin C and somewhat tasty.

Preparation: Infusion: Steep 6 tablespoons dried leaves in a quart of boiling hot water.

Contraindications: Do not use in large doses in pregnancy. The mild vasoconstricting property can constrict the capillary beds of uterus.

Uses/Dosage: One quart of the tea made with 6T of leaves a day
- Urinary tract disinfectant: Use for cystitis, urethritis, and long term low grade nephritis. Not enough for acute kidney infections.
- Sitz bath after birth or to treat hemorrhoids - combined with calendula, lavender, comfrey, and/or chamomile.

Combinations: The astringency may irritate the stomach lining, so consider combining with marshmallow root.

ARTEMISIA VULGARIS *Mugwort, Dreamweed*

Properties: Complex bitter, anti-inflammatory, strong antioxidant, overt liver stimulant, stimulates dreaming and psychic spaces.

Preparation: 1 tablespoon dry leaf per cup as a tea. Let steep 20 minutes.

Contraindications: Pregnancy or high flow menses. Can make migraines, allergies, arthritis worse. Increases inflammatory cascades.

Uses/Dosage: 1 tablespoon dry leaf per cup as a tea.
-Relaxes menstrual cramps and can bring on flow. Inhibits E-2 and F-2 prostaglandins which increase inflammation. Not a deep remedy, only for symptomatic relief of occasional discomfort.
- Bitter, stimulates digestion by reflex.
-Antioxidant: Will clear a frontal headache related to over indulging in fat within an hour. Drink the tea cold.
-Topical for anti-inflammatory, antibacterial. Can chew up and slap on wounds.
-For dreaming, mugwort can stimulates brighter, more memorable dreaming. Tends to bring up suppressed agendas, so good to add softening, nurturing herbs like chamomile, hops, lavender.

ASARUM *Wild Ginger*

Properties: Warming, diaphoretic, aromatic

Preparation: Use the whole plant as a fresh plant tincture. Rhizomes strongest. Fresh tincture 1:2; dry tincture 1:5 60% EtOH. A honey from the leaves for cough syrup is excellent.

Contraindications: Will make the uterus sweat, so avoid in pregnancy.

Uses/Dosage: 20-50 drops three times a day.
-To stimulate menstrual flow, especially when coming down with a cold at the same time.
-Digestive stimulant
-When flu is not resolving quickly enough, can use just a little.
-Aristolocheic acids dilate blood supply to central mesenteric and splanchnic arteries and dilate the periphery so you sweat more, and stimulate natural killer cells (NK cells) which scavenge dead and infected cells.

AVENA *Wild Oats*

Properties: Relaxes without sedation and without reducing mental clarity. Very distinct and wonderful remedy. Traditional nerve remedy.

Harvest: In the spring when seeds heads are in "milk" stage. i.e. the forming seed will exude a white milk when squeezed.

Preparation: Fresh plant tincture or glycerite.

Uses/Dosage: 1 dropperful to 1 teaspoon three times a day.
-Use in people that are hyper-mental. Is a gentle yin tonic to the nerves that calms the mind.

Combinations: Combine with ginseng or scutellaria (Skullcap).

BORAGO *Borage*

Properties: High in calcium and magnesium. Borage provides a sense of calming and being supported. Galactagogue.

Preparation: Simple infusion of the above ground parts of the plant. Borage oil is almost identical with evening primrose oil and usually less expensive.

Uses/Dosage: 1/2 to 1 oz of dry plant (above ground portion)
- Good generic tea for PMS: equal parts borage, chamomile, nettles and raspberry leaf.
- Boosts milk production because of its nutritive and calming properties.
- Good for menopause with blues, slight sense of heart palpations, and/or slight sense of warmth (not quite a hot flash).

CALENDULA OFFICINALIS

Properties: Anti-inflammatory. Antibacterial. Vulnerary - stimulates the growth of new tissue.

Preparation:
- Oil: powder dry flowers that have been slightly moistened with alcohol, then mix with oil. Use 1 ounce herb to 6 ounces oil. Use the oil to make salves.
- Tea: simmer 1 ounce herb in 1 quart water for 20 minutes
- Can mix powdered herbs into cocoa butter to prepare vaginal suppositories.

Uses/Dosage:
- Good topical for wound healing
- Use on burns, abrasions, diaper rash, sores on mucosa.
- Very sore nipples.
- Use in vaginal and cervical suppositories for ulcerations and inflammations
- Ok for chronic gastritis (common with hangover) (chamomile is better)

Combinations: With white sage for bacterial vaginitis or with Chilopsis for vaginal *Candida*.

CAPSELLA BURSA PASTORIS *Shepherd's purse, peppergrass*

Properties: Hemostatic. Mild oxytocin synergist.

Preparation: - Fresh plant tincture of above ground portion.

Uses/Dosage: Use 5-20 drops every 15-20 minutes for an hour.
- Most common use is for uterine passive hemorrhage. If this does not work, use another remedy like fresh trillium or compound tinctures of cinnamon and erigeron oils.
- Used in postpartum hemorrhage, post abortion excessive bleeding, uterine fibroid bleeding, endometrial bleeding, break-through bleeding, bleeding at ovulation, bleeding with Depo-Provera, prolonged spotting with IUD's, and ulcerative colitis.
-Can be used it menstrual flow is slow or fading in and out, this is good.

CAULOPHYLLUM *Blue Cohosh*

Properties: Oxytocin synergist

Preparation: Dry rhizome/root 1:5 in 65% alcohol

Contraindications: Do not use in pregnancy.

Uses/Dosage: 5-20 drops
- Any uterine conditions that are characterized by low oxytocin and loss of tone and structure.
- Can be used for menstrual cramping in low estrogen situations or to clarify menses. Start taking a few days before the period starts.

CHILOPSIS *Desert Willow*

Properties: Good antifungal: kills *Candida.*
Preparation: Tea made from 10 to 20 leaves per quart water. Steep the infusion 20 minutes. Suppository/bolus made from the powdered leaf in cocoa butter.

Uses/Dosage: Use a cup or two of the tea per day for *Candida* infections.
- Use suppository for vaginal yeast infections.

CIMICIFUGA RACEMOSA *Black Cohosh*
Black Cohosh, a plant indigenous to hardwood forests of the Eastern United States enjoys a wide range of use. Black Cohosh (Cimicifuga racemosa) is used extensively in Europe during menopause as a alternative to Estrogen Replacement Therapy (ERT). In America, its use has escalated due to the increased numbers of women seeking alternatives to ERT and the introduction and marketing of Remifemin (a German proprietary extract). It is claimed to be

beneficial in arthritis, muscle spasms, premenstrual syndrome, menstrual irregularities, and some types of headaches.

The effectiveness of Black Cohosh (BC) to alleviate the discomfort experienced at menopause has been investigated. It has been shown to reduce the frequency of hot flashes, a complaint of 75% of women undergoing the climacteric. In addition, clinical studies have demonstrated extracts of BC lessen the neurovegetative symptoms (moodiness, anxiety, depression) experienced at menopause.

Since its actions are similar to estrogen it was originally thought to be a phytoestrogen. More recent research has demonstrated that it has no estrogenic effects and instead acts on serotonin receptors.[4] My own research completed in 2000 suggested that *Cimicifuga* exerts its effect directly on the hypothalamus and not on the pituitary.

Recent research from Germany has shown black cohosh to have the same effect as HRT (conjugated estrogens) on menopausal symptoms and bone markers.[4] In studies that looked specifically at vaginal dryness, the vaginal mucosa improved after 12 weeks of treatment with Cimicifuga.[5]

Properties: Mimics estrogen in the body.

Preparation: Dry rhizome 1:5 70% alcohol. Powdered in capsules. Standardized extract are also available.

Contraindications: Do not use in pregnancy or bradykinin excess. Too large a dose can induce a frontal headache. It is a CNS depressant for some.

Uses/Dosage: Recommended dose: 40 - 1000 mg rhizome (10 to 25 drops tincture) to three times a day. Standardized extract (Remifemin®) use as directed.
- Works as well as estrogen replacement therapy for menopausal symptoms
- Helps with dull and heavy pain especially in the joints or menstrual cramping that feels like this.
- Use everywhere estrogen appears low and you want to juice things up.

CINNAMONUM *Cinnamon*

Properties: Warming, raises energy, decreases inflammation, hemostatic, carminative and spasmolytic..

Preparation: As a hemostat: Buy HerbPharm: Erigeron & Cinnamon Compound (6.25% cinnamon oil and 6.25% erigeron oil in alcohol.)

Uses/Dosage: As a hemostat: 5 drops every 15 minutes.
-- Used in postpartum hemorrhage, post abortion excessive bleeding, uterine fibroid bleeding, endometrial bleeding, break-through bleeding, bleeding at ovulation, bleeding with Depo-Provera, prolonged spotting with IUD's, and ulcerative colitis.
-Tea is astringent. It stimulates and calms digestion and helps stop diarrhea. Stimulates enzymes for better protein digestion. Enhances trypsin secretion.
- Clinical picture: cold on inside and edges, sores heal slowly, they don't repair quickly, slow, inflammation stays and perpetuates, vital forces are down, often see "runaway" inflammations or inflammations which have dragged on and become edematous. Good for these people.

CRYSANTHEMUM PARTHENIUM *Feverfew, Tanacetum, Pyrethrum*

Preparation: Fresh plant tincture, fresh plant

Uses/Dosage: 30 to 90 drops one to four times a day or one leaf a day to prevent migraines.
- Appears to strengthen/stabilize capillary beds. Use all month long for reduction/elimination of menstrual migraines.

DIOSCOREA VILLOSA *Wild Yam*
People claim this plant is converted to progesterone in the body. This simply is not true. Wild yam can serve as a precursor to progesterone that is synthesized in the laboratory or factory, but the body makes progesterone from cholesterol and the compounds in wild yam will not do. Still,

women report a progesterone like activity (which has not been scientifically validated) when using wild yam. After years of arguing with my health care practitioners I finally tried wild yam for my menstrual migraines. Internal use of tincture didn't do anything, but when I used it topically I got the "progestogenic" effect people were talking about. I propose that there are compounds in the plant that interact with progesterone receptors or with the progesterone signaling system to mimic progesterone and/or potentiate the effects of progesterone. In addition, it is possible that this effect may only be observable in human and not in the animal models used in science.

Properties: Antispasmodic in smooth muscle (tubular organs: intestines, stomach, gallbladder, uterus). Mimics progesterone.

Preparation: Tincture rhizome 1:5 in 60% alcohol. Oil extract of rhizome 1:5 or 1:6

Contraindications:

Uses/Dosage: Recommended dose: topical application of 100-1000 mg rhizome in the form of 3-6 sprays tincture or ¼ t. oil daily throughout the cycle.
- Use wild yam (topical application) in situations where progesterone seems low.
- Wild yam is also a nice smooth muscle relaxant. Take internally to relieve nausea, morning sickness, intestinal cramping, and menstrual cramping.

ELEUTHEROCOCCUS *Siberian Ginseng*

Properties: Adaptogenic. This has neutral energy - compare to American Ginseng which is cooling and Chinese Ginseng which is warming.

Preparation: 1:1 fluid extract or purchase standardized 5:1 or 10:1 extract (dry). Most standardized extracts are comparable. Imperial Elixir is the brand I use. It has a great price. They market several versions which are actually identical but marketed to different people. Right now Siberian Sport 5000 has the best price on Amazon. The label is marked

Uses/Dosage: 1 dropper to 1 tsp three times a day of fluid extract. 1 to 4 capsules (equivalent to 2.5 to 10 grams of whole root) per day
- All purpose herb for supporting the body's capacity for dealing with stress.

- Improves memory and ability to perform.
- May act as a stimulant for the first few days, then it is neutral.
- Modulates the adrenal system and the immune system in particular.
- Appropriate for most everybody and can be used long term.
- Improves recovery from labor.

ERIGERON CANADENSE *Canadian Fleabane*

Properties: Warming astringent, hemostatic with focus on intestines and uterus. Very peppery taste: If you bite it, it "bites" back.

Preparation: As a hemostat: Buy HerbPharm: Erigeron & Cinnamon Compound (6.25% cinnamon oil and 6.25% erigeron oil in alcohol.)

Uses/Dosage: As a hemostat: 5 drops every 15 minutes.
-- Used in postpartum hemorrhage, post abortion excessive bleeding, uterine fibroid bleeding, endometrial bleeding, break-through bleeding, bleeding at ovulation, bleeding with Depo-Provera, prolonged spotting with IUD's, and ulcerative colitis.

FOUQUERIA SPLENDENS *Ocotillo*

Properties: Ocotillo gets better absorption of fats and oils by stimulating better movement of pelvic lymph.

Preparation: Fresh tincture of inner and outer bark. Pick older ocotillo with less thorns. Pound stem with a rock to remove bark.

Uses/Dosage: Two dropperfuls up to four times a day
Useful in:
- Pelvic congestion. Heaviness or fullness in pelvis. Tired legs.

- Portal hypertension causing hemorrhoids or varicose veins.
- Ovarian cysts. Combine with *Ceonothus*.
- After successful treatment of Pelvic Inflammatory Disease (PID) (chlamydia) when there is still swelling.
- Difficulty handling fats, i.e. tired after high fat meal, maybe with spots in front of the eyes.
- Will help with bleeding fibroids.

Combinations: Combine with *Collinsonia* for better venous tone.

GARRYA *Silk Tassel*

Garrya is an evergreen bush which can be found growing at the California coast as well as in the dry mountains and foothills.

Properties: Anticholinergic. (Small amounts of acetylcholine act as muscle relaxant, high amounts cause muscle spasm.)

Part Used: In order of increasing strength: leaf, twig, root, root bark

Preparation: Fresh plant tincture or dry plant tincture in 75% alcohol.

Uses/Dosage: The leaf tincture is used at 2 -3 dropperfuls. The root bark is dosed at 5-15 drops. This plant is used as one might use aspirin, only when needed. It is not a tonic! The therapeutic dose and the side effect producing dose are close. Side effects: cold, clammy, flushed face, dilated pupils, etc.
- *Garrya* is a smooth muscle relaxant. Best results are obtained when used for severe cramping of smooth muscles. This includes tissue such as intestines (Crohn's disease, ulcerative colitis, or other inflammatory intestinal condition), uterus (menstrual cramps), ureters (passing kidney stones), and bile duct (gall bladder attack or gallstones).

Combinations: Good to support with milder antispasmodics: Catnip, wild yam, cramp bark, or homeopathic magnesium phos.

GELSEMIUM SEMPERVIRENS *Yellow Jasmine*

Properties: Narcotic

Harvest: Autumn

Preparation: Fresh root/rhizome tincture. Or purchase homeopathic.

Contraindications: Pregnancy and lactation. Hypotension, bradycardia other disease states.

Uses/Dosage: Put one drop in a quart of water and sip. For most people 1 drop is more than enough. Dangerous in large doses. Try the homeopathic for the same results.
- Lessens tension in the meninges and lining of the brain. Wards off oncoming migraines in prodromal stage. *Predictable.* Often as little as 1/10 of a drop will stop the process. Will work within minutes.

GOSSYPIUM *Wild Cotton*

Properties: Oxytocin mimetic.

Preparation: Fresh root bark tincture.

Contraindications: Pregnancy. Not safe to use in women long term.

Uses/Dosage: 15-45 drops to four times a day.
-Good for menstruation or ovulation which fade in and out. Improves corpus luteum formation (CL compromised in unclear or late starting menses).
- Good for women prone to ectopic pregnancy. Gets better movement of eggs through the fallopian tubes.
- Increases lactation in low oxytocin pattern.
- For swollen breasts use Gossypium a few days before expected menses.
- For secondary amenorrhea give this around/at ovulation. (Simulate cycle using estrogen agonist and Vitex)

Combinations: Use with an estrogen mimetic.

LEONORUS *Motherwort*

Properties: Reduces thyroid hormones, GnRH, LH and FSH.

Preparation: Fresh plant tincture

Contraindications: Avoid in pregnancy. May push a perimenopausal woman back to having menses again. In high estrogen types it can create excessive flow.

Uses/Dosage: Use 10 to 30 dropperfuls to three times a day.

- Use whenever you feel the need for "mothering".
- Strongly reduces thyroid hormones and production of LH and FSH.
- Heart palpitations, or irregular heart beat.
- Use 5 to 20 drops in a cup of water sipped throughout the day for post-partum depression that follows the progesterone drop after childbirth.
- Perimenopausal depression and hot flashes with the blues. Good for this, but *Lycopus* is superior by far.
- PMS with lots of moodiness and cramping.
- Can be used to bring on period. Will relieve cramps and increase flow.

LOBELIA INFLATA *Pukeweed*

Properties: General parasympathetic mimetic, entire system, not just vagus nerve.

Preparation: Fresh plant tincture 1:5 instead of 1:2 (Alkaloids precipitate out if stronger.)

Uses/Dosage: Use five to 20 drops. Too much may cause nausea.
- As parasympathetic mimetic, it is good for everything from asthma to premature ejaculation.
- Will relax the sharp edge of nearly spasmodic muscle contraction in uterus as well as relax the cervical os, great for pain of miscarriage. Use frequent doses.
- Sometimes with poor fluid movement through uterus due to sympathetic excess, there can be heavy cramping or sluggish menses. Lobelia is good for this.

Combinations: With *Lycopus* and or *Anemone* for hot flashes

---

LYCOPUS *Bugleweed*

Properties: Decreases thyroid functions. Works very fast and systemically, both via brain (produce less TRH and TSH) and via body (use less thyroid hormone). Will see most effect at juncture of thyroid and lungs.

Preparation: Fresh plant tincture.

Uses/Dosage: 10 to 30 drops up to four times a day.
- High thyroid symptoms: speedy metabolism, all the way through the body they will burn hot and fast, sleepless, increased rate of respiration and heart beat (tachycardia as well as palpitations and arrhythmias), mind spinning hard, tissue repair is rapid, often rapid GI transit time. Pulse is fast but not strong. After awhile there is a hollow energetic, false fire. Thyroid stress pattern is common, it is a stress manipulation like adrenaline stress pattern.
- Menopausal hot flashes. This reduces GnRH. Many connections between thyroid and gonadal functions. Lycopus is safe gentle herb here, no problems like with Leonurus.
- Osteogenesis imperfecta- when this is coupled with hyperthyroid, Lycopus can help. These people have high need for minerals but no appetite, so they leach calcium from bones.
- Not useful for Hashimotos' thyroid which is an autoimmune attack on thyroid.

Combinations: Mix with *Lobelia* and *Anemone* as appropriate.

MAHONIA *Oregon Grape, Berberis*

Properties: Yellow bitter. Liver stimulant. Immune stimulant. Antibiotic.

Preparation: Fresh plant tincture.

Contraindications: Do not use with western medications. The yellow bitters tend to complicate Western medications, changing the speed with which they are broken down or removed from the body. This is seen especially with sulfa drugs and the tricyclics of the 2nd, 3rd, and 4th generations.

Uses/Dosage: 15-30 drops several times each day.
- Digestive stimulant - use a dropperful before eating. Aids in the digestion of fats and oils.
- Stimulates liver to be more anabolic. Broad spectrum herb for liver deficiency. Liver clears inflammatory complexes from blood. So, *Mahonia* will help with chronic inflammations in liver deficiency people.
- Good for poorly healing skin/mucosa. Good support for clearing hay fever, asthma, eczema, and all allergic responses.
- Helps deal with die off of major *Candida* blooms and leaky gut syndrome.

Combinations: If low thyroid consider ginseng/*Centella*. If low reproductive consider *Angelica sinensis*.

MEDICAGO *Alfalfa*
Research has shown that these alfalfa plants communicate via sound waves. If you pick half a field the remaining plants will become bitter. Thinking they used chemical messengers to communicate, researchers isolated the plants. They remaining plants still turned bitter.

Properties: Diuretic, high in calcium, phosphorous, and magnesium, alterative.

Preparation: Tea - simple infusion. 1ounce dried plant to 1 quart water.

Uses/Dosage: Use as needed. Alfalfa helps alkalinize the blood so it carries waste better. Gentle supportive herb.

MELALEUCA *Tea tree*
Two species: tea tree and cajaput. To herbalists they are about the same, to aromatherapists they are quite different.

Properties: Strong antibacterial and antifungal.

Preparation: Essential oil.

Uses/Dosage:
- Bacterial vaginosis- suppositories made with 2-3 drops of oil per suppository.

NEPETA *Catnip*

Properties: Bitter. GI stimulant. Calms stomach, uterus. Promotes menstrual flow.

Preparation: Dry plant tincture 50% alcohol or fresh plant tincture.

Contraindications: Do not use in pregnancy.

Uses/Dosage:
- Safe for little kids, and strong enough for adults. In kids it will break fevers, and in both kids and adults it is strongly relaxing, and relieves digestive tract spasm all the way through stomach and small intestine and reflex spasm in large intestine. Not for ulcerative colitis pain. Settles upset stomach.
- Very good with bad menstrual cramps.   Will slightly increase flow.
- Small amounts are good for nausea in pregnancy, but do not use if there is any history of miscarriage.

NUPHAR LUTEA *Yellow Pond Lily*.

Properties: Cooling, quieting.

Preparation: -Fresh plant tincture. Powdered, in bolus, for cervix.

Uses/Dosage: Dose is high, 60 drops and work up to 1/2 teaspoon.
- Can be very good with ovarian and fallopian tube pain. Hot and irritated.
- Uterine -hot, swollen or boggy, and irritated with excessive flow.
- Irritated cervix. Use powdered in bolus applied to cervix and tincture orally. Brings down

inflammation and checks excessive flow. Regain tissue integrity. With any STD, you want to get better tissue integrity as well as kill the agent of infection.

- Many women claim it works with excessive flow which goes on far too long.

Combinations: Bacterial vaginitis salve: cocoa butter base. Finely powdered Nuphar, calendula, white sage, and tea tree oil. Make small boluses, and, once hard, dip in successive layers of cocoa butter until they have a smooth finish. Before inserting, hold in hand or in pocket to bring close to body temperature.

ONEOTHERA *Evening Primrose*

Properties: Anti-inflammatory. Contains GLA.

Preparation: -Tea of entire above ground plant. Oil.

Uses/Dosage:

- Changes arachidonic acid cascades, resulting in less spasm and inflammation. Many of the body's inflammatory responses will respond well to this. Certain eicosanoids get platelets to stick together. This can help some people with thick, sticky blood to avoid hardening of arteries.

- Brain effects. A woman's brain needs estrogen. Too much or too little makes them feel bad. Evening Primrose oil is good for women who feel dreadful mood swings with PMS, and will lead to a period with far less cramping. Estrogen increases menstrual cramps. This stops that. Very good when doubled over with pain, puking, and sensitive to light. Sometimes migraines are a part of this picture, too. It may helps with them also.

- Mastalgia. Take internally. Premenstrual mastalgia, pain from fibrocystic breasts- will slow down the growth and pain. Add fresh plant tincture of whole violet plant.

- Rheumatoid and osteo arthritis - can be amazing. Don't be afraid to use a lot, this is a safe plant. Judy Beaver knows a woman who transplanted a lot into her garden so she would have plenty to make tea from. Cleared up her advanced rheumatoid arthritis.

Combinations: Use with fresh plant tincture of entire violet plant for fibrocystic breasts.

PHYTOLACCA *Pokeroot*

Properties: Immune stimulant. Mitogen. Strong macrophage stimulator- activity and proliferation. Strong action in any area with lots of lymph cells (throat, breast).

Preparation: - Fresh tincture.

Contraindications: Fairly toxic. Use to get things started. Don not use in acute conditions like new cold or flu. Use cautiously or will make people feel like they have the flu: sore joints, nausea.

Uses/Dosage: Under 5 drops of tincture.
- Skin infections, tonsillitis, mastitis.
- After menses sometimes women get really swollen lymph nodes in their armpits. This is very good for that. Helps break down extra proteins stuck in lymph system.
- Used primarily as kicker when immune system is not working well and you want to rev it up.
- Acute infections or long term infections which are not resolving.

PIPER METHYSTICUM *Kava Kava*

Properties: Smooth muscle relaxant.

Preparation: Fresh root tincture is best, but dry will work. 1:5 75% alcohol. Or use standardized extract.
-Mashed root simmered in coconut milk is traditional preparation for ceremonies and dream work.

Uses/Dosage:
- Relieves menstrual cramps.
- Urinary tract pain- pain on urination- numbs.
- Sometimes helps with urethral stricture. Use with Gelsemium. Stricture feels like infection, but when get blood work up - no elevation in white blood cell count.

RUBUS IDAEUS *Red Raspberry, Black Raspberry*

Properties: Rose family astringent. Contains Ca, Mg, Fe.

Preparation: Make tea from leaf or root bark. Make tea with 1 oz per quart.

Uses/Dosage: Use 1 to 4 cups of the tea a day.
- Slightly decreases menstrual flow. May help with menstrual cramps.
- Relaxes uterus and yet gives better tone to uterine muscles. Give all the way through pregnancy, not just in the last trimester. Everything goes better, quicker labor, though not harsh or too quick; does not produce fetal distress. When drinking same thing every bloody day, can get awful tired of it, so switch to nettle tea sometimes, but as much as possible during pregnancy, drink this every day.

SALVIA APIANA *White Sage*

Properties: Cosmic incense plant/good smudge. Astringent, antibacterial, slows secretions in certain mucous membranes, reduces lactation.

Preparation: Put in salves or suppositories. Burn as incense. Make into tea.

Uses/Dosage:
- Good bolus (with slippery elm and tea tree oil) for bacterial vaginosis.
- Good gargle for sore throat, tonsillitis. 1/3 cup vinegar, 2/3 cup hot sage tea, and a couple grinds of black pepper from a mill. Gargle 1 mouthful at a time and spit out.
- Good rinse for gum infections
- Good hair rinse
- Reduces lactation.

Combinations: With slippery elm, calendula, and tea tree oil for bacterial vaginosis

SCUTELLARIA *Scullcap*

Properties: Mildly sedating, relaxing, significant anti-inflammatory nervine.

Preparation: -Fresh plant tincture of above ground plant. Wild varieties are stronger than the domestic variety.

Uses/Dosage:

-Relaxing. Stress falls down and off the body leaving the mind alert. Perfect for test taking. Quality is cooling, people feel like nerves are nourished, insulated, more flexible.

- Sometimes will work with headaches. Take at night when you think you might wake up with a headache. Constant use may result in less severe and less frequent migraines. Occasionally too much can bring on headaches.

- Late menses due to stress- 5 to 10 drops can bring on menses quickly.

- Good for tremors.

- Very large amounts can help people through withdrawal.

- PMS moodiness: combine with avena, celery seed, lavender, hypericum.

Note: Daily use can result in the body developing tolerance. You may need to increase your dose over time. To recalibrate body, just do not use it for a couple of days and the response will become sensitive again.

Combinations: HerbPharm Avena Skullcap Combination is very nice for PMS stress.

SERENOA REPENS *Saw Palmetto*

Properties: Mild but noticeable anabolic steroid agonist. Juices you up, changes the way the body processes hormones.

Preparation: -Lots of standardized extracts on market, they probably all work.

Uses/Dosage:

- Can increase seminal fluid quantity and quality.

- - Effective treatment for benign prostatic hyperplasia (BPH).   More effective than pharmaceuticals. Serenoa helps reduce swelling which can cause lack of force of urination, dribbling, and pain after or with orgasm.

- Low sex drive in men with dry throat and reduced ejaculate.

- Can help with dry cervical mucosa. Lack of ferning. Low estrogen or poor estrogen use will produce lack of ferning. This is often from subclinical low thyroid. Combine with estrogen agonist for estrogen boost.

- Boggy uterine tissue

- Menopausal dry throat

STELLARIA MEDIA *Chickweed*

Chickweed looks a lot like scarlet pimpernel which is toxic. Scarlet pimpernel has milky sap, red flower, and no fur. Chickweed does not have milky sap, has a white flower, and has fur up one side of the stem, often switching sides.

Properties: Cooling. Diuretic.

Preparation: Tasty addition to salads. Fresh plant tincture.

Uses/Dosage: Use 2 dropperfuls (over time) for menopausal hot flashes.

TARAXACUM *Dandelion*

Identification: True dandelion: flower heads never branch, leaves all form basal rosette - no branching, flower stem is tubular and has milky sap, leaves smooth - not hairy.

Properties Very high in vitamins A, C, E, K, and minerals; 1 oz dry leaf has more vitamin C than 2 cup orange juice. Leaf is strong diuretic fresh or dry. Dry root is primarily focused on the liver, fresh root has direct systemic effects as well as liver focus. Cooling herb.

Preparation: Fresh leaf tincture, fresh leaf as food, or dry leaf tea is strong a diuretic. Fresh leaves at grocery store are not true dandelion leaves. Dry root decoct up to 1 oz dry herb per day or use capsules. 3-6 caps per day of freeze dried root (Eclectic institute). Also, can just chew on the fresh root, just a little piece three times a day. Too much is mildly laxative.

Uses/Dosage

Leaf

- Strong diuretic. Big handful of dry leaf in pot, steep for a long time.
- Commonly used with UTI's when want to dilute the urine to change the pH to make less hospitable to invading organisms.
- Edema. Safe general herb for edema. Strong but gentle.

Root

- Dry root is straight up simple bitter, not like the yellow bitters. This is strong anti-inflammatory to liver and clears waste, increases bile production. May also push lymph out of liver, and so get more waste out. Shrinks liver inflammation very well.
- Will relieve jaundice (from virus or solvents) rapidly: reversal in 24-48 hours. 1 oz root simmered as decoction; 2 cups three times a day. Stick with it for about 2 weeks or it will return. The liver is swollen and this shuts the bile duct, so the bile shunts into general circulation. Intestinal regulation requires bile to work properly, so this will improve digestion when there is jaundice, such as the abdominal malaise attendant to hepatitis.
- Helps secrete uric acid- joint pain decreases. Good arthritis herb.
- Fresh root long term for anabolic excess constitution with allergies and/or menopausal hot flashes.
- Improved liver anti inflammatory response. When the liver is inflamed, there is a shift in what the liver produces. Acute phase proteins are probably the first immune protein response, and there is a change in the lipids produced- more LDL's and VLDL's which are used as fuel normally but when produced in excess, they get more incorporated into cell membranes and this increases inflammatory responses.
- Very good for creating a positive shift in cholesterol levels.
- Fresh root has more action as systemic anti inflammatory - primarily liver, skin, and joints. One of the best treatments for hives. 2 caps three times a day.

THUJA *Western red cedar*

Properties: Green leaves are a great incense combined with osha. Antiviral, antifungal, antibacterial; some tissue specificity to lung, somewhat secreted by kidneys. Immune stimulant-

macrophages and NK cells.

Preparation: Essential oil, fresh leaf tincture
Contraindications: Do not use in pregnancy

Uses/Dosage: Primary use is topical antifungal.
- For athletes foot, put in spray bottle and spray several times/day, and change socks daily.
- Very good for warts (antiviral and increases macrophage and NK scavenging). For hand/foot warts try cauterization followed by application of essential oil. Works very well. They don't come back.
- Human Papilloma Virus (HPV) more than 1/3 of college women have it, at UC Berkley it is about 80%. Often on both internal and external genitalia, thighs, anal tissue. Soak a tampon in a solution of a teaspoon of tincture in a few oz of water, insert and remove the applicator. Could possibly make a spray work. There is a specific strain of HPV which leads to very increased rate of cervical cancer, it can be tested for.   Men can contract and carry HPV. Getting people out of blame patterns about where they got HPV is important. It can stay dormant for decades before it shows up. It is like trying to figure out where you got herpes when you have many partners.

TRIFOLIUM PRATENSE *Red Clover, White Clover*

Properties: Gentle, for lungs and skin. Alkalinizes blood, increases carrying capacity for wastes. Mild blood cooler. High in minerals

Preparation: Whole bud, should be reddish purple make into a simple infusion. Standardized Extract: Promensil. 500mg tablet has 40 mg isoflavones. 1gram dry clover contains about 20mg isoflavones.[20]

Uses/Dosage:
- Gentle support tea for people facing skin eruptions, eczema, hives.
- Nice support for fasting, since there is an increase of acidic wastes at this time.
- Supportive for chemotherapy; helps with the extra waste generated.
- Use this when the person is not eating, and is sweating a lot with fever, and the tongue gets funky, bad smelling, acrid. Usually they smell terrible, bad enough you want to open a window.
- When you want to work on liver but can't because the person is on pharmaceuticals use this.

TRILLIUM *Bethroot or Birthroot.*

Properties: Oxytocinergic (does not have oxytocin but amplifies bodies response to it.) When other stop-capillary-bed-hemorrhaging remedies fail, use this.

Preparation: Fresh root tincture Fresh leaf tincture is effective also, use higher dose. Pick leaves after seeding so as not to disturb reproduction.

Uses/Dosage: Fresh root tincture 5-10 drops(large dose can increase bleeding). Fresh leaf tincture - about 20-30 drops.
- A little works to stop capillary bed hemorrhaging, too much stimulates more blood flow. Used after childbirth, abortion.
- Bleeding fibroids- take dose more frequently.
- Start/stop menses is often poor oxytocin response. Big stress often reduces oxytocin production. Usually it is poor estrogen setup, though- estrogen sets up oxytocin receptor sites.
- Nosebleed- oxytocin will contract capillary beds anywhere.

URTICARIA *Nettles*

Properties: Food plant: 10% protein by weight, rich in Ca, Mg, Fe, Vit A, C, K. Diuretic. Hemostatic. Anti-inflammatory.

Preparation: Dry as tea or powdered in capsules. Fresh tincture and fresh freeze dried capsules. Great as cream of nettles soup.

Contraindications: Pregnancy in Indian women.

Uses/Dosage: 2 to 6 fresh freeze dried caps as needed for allergies. Works within 1/2 hour. Can prevent allergies for the season if you start at the beginning of the season.
- With raspberry for excessive uterine bleeding.
- General hemostatic for either acute irritation (nosebleed) or congestion with ulceration.
- Great pregnancy tea (see contraindication above).

VIBURNUM OPULUS *Cramp Bark, High Cranberry Bush*

Properties: Works primarily on uterine cramps and areas with similar nerve nexus in the lower abdomen.

Preparation: Dry root bark tincture 1:4 in 60% alcohol. Steep 20 minutes or more for the tea.

Uses/Dosage: 1-3 droppers full of tincture as needed. 1 teaspoon to 1 Tablespoon per cup tea.
- For many women, this alone will clear menstrual cramps.
- Abortion/extraction/early miscarriage cramps. Can even arrest a miscarriage. Estrogens levels are relatively high in pregnancy and oxytocin responds to it. HCG's and progesterone should be balancing the spasm producing aspect of the estrogen. Use viburnum in vast amounts in painful miscarriage, it will not interfere with the uterus's normal ability to clear itself, the normal (non-spasming) push will continue. Atropine and others *will* interfere.
- High estrogen/low progesterone type constitution will show symptoms like: nausea, cramping, heavy flow, premenstrual migraines. When you see a miscarriage with this history, there is a chance you can arrest it.

Combinations: - Mix in Nuphar to slow down cervical flow better.

Notes: Viburnum prunifolia (Black Haw) is used the same way.

VITEX AGNUS-CASTUS *Chaste Tree Berries, Monk's Pepper*
Grows great in Phoenix.

Premenstrual syndrome (PMS) has been shown to effect up to 3-5% of women in their reproductive years. The reason for this condition is multifactorial, of which stress and diet may have a role. A significant percentage of visits to the primary care physician are related to this condition. Allopathic treatments include hormonal therapy, antidepressants and diuretics. These treatments have on occasion significant adverse effects, and rarely severe complications.

Vitex is an alternative to prescription drug treatment for premenstrual syndrome (PMS) or menstrual disorders. It has been shown to effectively treat mastodynia, water retention, acne vulgaris, depression, anxiety, cravings, and luteal phase defects in clinical trials conducted in Germany.[21,22,23,24]

Several compounds in vitex bind to dopamine receptors and act to decrease prolactin.[25,26] It is elevated prolactin (or increased prolactin release with stress) that is thought to lead to luteal phase defects. The proposed mechanism of action is supported by the observed clinical results. In addition, vitex has also been used to help curb cravings at detoxification clinics. Again due to its dopamine effects.

Vitex has a rich traditional use for over 2000 years, first recorded by Hippocrates 400 BC. Presently Vitex is most commonly used by European physicians for various menstrual disorders, including PMS, and approved by the Commission E, in Germany. Over the last 50 years there have been a substantial number of studies on Vitex, especially in Germany to understand the mechanism of action. As a whole plant there are many constituents such as diterpenes, flavonoids, and irridoid glycosides that act, possibly synergistically, in an indirect way on various neurotransmitters and hormones. Vitex effects the dominergic (D2) receptors in the pituitary by inhibiting/modulating the release of prolactin, and thus influencing the progesterone/luteal phase of the menstrual cycle. More recent studies show that hormone, opioid and acetylcholine receptor sites may be effected.

Properties: Dopamine agonist, reduces prolactin, increases LH.

Preparation: Tincture 1:5 60% alcohol

Uses/Dosage: 40 – 1000 mg berry (20 drops tincture) to three times a day

- Increases and stabilized the hypothalamic process of increasing LH levels, which will in the short run increase progesterone levels. Picture: menses very crampy, sugar craving, premenstrual migraines, thin flow. If trying to stop miscarriage give twice daily.
- If low estrogen and low progesterone type, give this, it will set up better estrogen sites because they begin with progesterone. (Each gives rise to the other, and estrogen makes receptor sites for oxytocin) Estrogen is catabolic but looks anabolic, progesterone is more anabolic.
- Can be used all month long or take one week before PMS begins: water retention, moodiness, profuse but thin, not thick and heavy flow. High progesterone menses is more characterized by thick and heavy flow and acne, especially in the groove below lower lip.
- Often very nice to even out gonadotropic menopausal symptoms, hot flashes and moodiness. Takes a while to work.
- Often brings on lactation well. Use with estrogen agonist.

Combinations: For PMS, try to get breakdown of hormones faster: Use Mahonia and something cooling to liver like burdock or dandelion.

WITHANIA SOMNIFERA *Ashwagandha, Indian ginseng*

Properties: Adaptogen, Anti-inflammatory, sedative (appears to mimic GABA), anti-oxidant, anti-fungal, immunomodulatory, smooth muscle relaxant, memory improvement, and cognition enhancing.

Preparation: Dry root powdered in capsules. Fresh or Dry root tincture.

Uses/Dosage: 1 to 2 dropperfuls to three times a day.

Adaptogens are plants that help the body "adapt" to stress. They help counteract the toll that living in the modern world takes on us. Using plants like Ashwagandha on a regular basis enhances one's ability to stay well. Ashwagandha is a well researched plant. It has been demonstrated to be very useful in relieving the symptoms of arthritis. It is also a mild sedative (so it the ginsengs are too stimulating for you then this plant may suit you well.) Although it seems to "cool out" the brain, it also enhances cognition and memory.

ZINGIBER *Ginger*

Properties: Clears nausea, carminative, slows gut transit time, mild liver protecting effects, anti-inflammatory, diaphoretic. Dry rhizome warms more inside; fresh rhizome increases sweat more.

Preparation: Decoction: use three quarter size slices to 12 ounces of water and simmer down to a cup of water. For morning sickness, candy made from ginger is often more user friendly.

Uses/Dosage:
- Stimulating to cephalic phase of digestion- gets everything which follows working better. Some people only need a little crystallized ginger before meals.
- Changes intestinal peristalsis. 2 primary motions: 1) forward- slows this down 2) churning- increases this. It does not slow digestion, it slows transit time while increasing churning.

- Nausea of any kind. Decreases motion sickness; better than Dramamine (US army study). Morning sickness in pregnancy, etc.

- Increases blood flow to abdomen.

- Increases menstrual flow a bit. Sometimes a single cup of ginger tea can reduce menstrual cramping.

BEYOND THE PHYSICAL

Long before cancer shows up as a tumor there is a blockage of energy in the spot. That is what I learned when I was seventeen and studying Traditional Chinese Medicine. Indeed, before any illness can manifest as a physical reality the energy flow through the area must be blocked. This is actually corroborated by western thought. Long before you have a tumor, at least five different systems must fail, such as one of the many cancer cells that arises each day in our bodies escaping detection by the immune system. In a sense, this represents a block in the smooth functioning of the body or a disruption in the energy flow.

My internal arts practice (chi gung, tai chi, etc) has taught me that the mind moves the energy (and conversely the energy can move the mind). Underneath the physical body is an energy body and underneath that is the mind controlling it all. The physical is a manifestation of our mind. While this treatise is focused on working with the physical body using physical means it is also possible to change the physical body by working directly with the mind. Even genetic diseases are ultimately under the control of our mind and can be changed. Our mind creates our world and even though the world seems fixed and solid, it is ultimately quite mutable.

In my book, *The Twelve Steps as a Path to Enlightenment - How the Buddha Works the Steps,* I describe the Buddhist model for the creation of the world. The ideas I present there are very much in line with what we know to be true from quantum physics. They key idea that is important to mention here is that what we believe to be true is not Ultimate Truth. Our beliefs can be quite arbitrary and unless we've taken the time to examine them, they can represent absurd or limiting ideas.

For instance, calling menstruation "the curse" is a sure fire way to create a cursed experience of our monthly cycle. Further, women with a history of sexual trauma are more apt to have conscious or subconscious beliefs regarding sexual safety, the value they hold as a woman, the worth of a woman's body, etc that can affect the flow of energy through the sexual organs and contribute to painful menses and organic disease. While herbs can support physical health, ultimately dysfunctional beliefs need to be rooted out and discarded.

Beliefs to check:

I love myself.

I hate myself.

Sex is enjoyable.

Sexual expression is safe.

It is safe to be a woman.

I love my body.

I hate my body.

My body heals easily

My body and I have a good relationship.

I listen to my body.

I respond to my body's needs.

I nurture my body.

I am cursed.

Cancer or another disease runs in my family.

I have my mother's _____

I am healthy.

I am sick.

I am beautiful.

I am sexy.

I am attractive.

I am powerful.

I am ugly.

It is safe to be beautiful.

I am ruined.

I am damaged goods.

I have to sacrifice my body for others.

I am cursed.

I have this disease to honor my mother, etc.

I love women.

I love men.

I hate women.

I hate men.

<u>Questions to help with the exploration of non-physical causes of dysfunction:</u>

Hey body, what are you trying to tell me?

Can I change this issue? Can I change it now? What would it take to change this issue now?

What is holding this disease/issue/problem in place?

What would happen if I was completely free from this issue now? What would I lose that having this gives me?

What physical actualization of a healthy, open, free, beautiful woman am I now capable of being?

What belief is holding this in place?

What am I disowning to hold this in place?

Hey body, what could we be doing if we weren't doing this?

How does this serve me?

When did this issue start? What was going on in my life at the time?

Hey body, do you want to take this drug/herb/supplement/food? How much? How often?

Will this drug/herb/supplement/food contribute to my body, being and/or life?

Is there something else I need to know?

Is there something that I am refusing to acknowledge or see?

What do I know that I am pretending not to know or denying that I know?

REFERENCES

Colleen O. Davis, Red Tape Tightrope: Regulating Financial Conflicts of Interest in FDA Advisory Committees, 91 WASH. U.L. Rev. 1591 (2014).

[2] John Kelley, Antidepressants: Do they "work" or don't they?, Scientific American, Mar2, 2010.

[3] Alving, B. *Statement on Oral Contraceptive Study from Barbara Alving, M.D., Director of the Women's Health Initiative and Acting Director of the National Heart, Lung, and Blood Institute.* [Press Release] 2004 Dec 15, 2004 [cited 2008 Dec 17]; Available from: http://www.nhlbi.nih.gov/new/press/04-12-15.htm.

[4] NCI. *FactSheet for Oral Contraceptives and Cancer Risk.* 2006 5/4/2006 [cited 2008 Dec 17]; Available from: http://www.cancer.gov/cancertopics/factsheet/Risk/oral-contraceptives. Updated: 2012.

[5]Shaw, C.R. 1997. The perimenopausal hot flash: epidemiology, physiology, and treatment. Nurse Practitioner, 22:3, 55-6, 61-6.

[6] Merchenthaler, I., J.M. Funkhouser, J.M. Carver, S.G. Lundeen, K Ghosh, and R.C. Winneker, 1998. The effect of estrogens and antiestrogens in a rat model for hot flush. Maturitas, 30:3, 307-316.

[7] Lieberman, S. 1998. A review of the effectiveness of Cimicifuga racemosa (Black Cohosh) for the symptoms of menopause. Journal of Women's Health, 7:5, 525-529.

[8] Liske, E. 1998. Therapeutic efficacy and safety of *Cimicifuga racemosa* for gynecologic disorders. Advances in Therapy 15:1, 45-53.

[9] Liske, E. 1998, Therapy of Climacteric Complaints with Cimicifuga racemosa: herbal medicine with clinically proven evidence. Menopause, 5:4, 250.

[10] Mielnik, J. 1997. Extract of Cimicifuga racemosa in the treatment of neurovegetative symptoms in women in the perimenopausal period. Maturitas, 27:Suppl., 215.

[11] NIH, *Facts about menopausal hormone therapy.* 2005, National Institutes of Health: Washington, D.C. p. 1-24.

[12] http://lifeissues.net/writers/wilks/wilks_06hormonaldruguse.html Accessed Oct 3, 2015.

[13] Geller, S.E. and L. Studee, *Botanical and dietary supplements for menopausal symptoms: what works, what does not.* J Womens Health (Larchmt), 2005. **14**(7): p. 634-49.

[14] Trickey, R., *Women, Hormones and the Menstrual Cycle.* 1998, Australia: Allen & Unwin. 503.

[15] Smith, C.J., *Non-Hormonal Control of Vaso-Motor Flushing in Menopausal Patients.* Chicago Medicine, 1964.

[16] Kerstetter JE(1), Mitnick ME, Gundberg CM, Caseria DM, Ellison AF, Carpenter TO, Insogna KL., *Changes in bone turnover in young women consuming different levels of dietary protein.* J Clin Endocrinol Metab. 1999

Mar;84(3):1052-5.

[17] Schwalfenberg, G. K. (2012). The Alkaline Diet: Is There Evidence That an Alkaline pH Diet Benefits Health? *Journal of Environmental and Public Health, 2012*, 727630. http://doi.org/10.1155/2012/727630

[18] http://nof.org/faq/588 National Osteoporosis Foundation accessed 3Oct2015.

[19] https://www.drfuhrman.com/library/diet_soda_deplete_calcium_from_bone.aspx#_ENREF_3 Accessed 3Oct 2015.

[20]USDA, *USDA-Iowa State University Database on the Isoflavone Content of Foods.* 2002, U.S. Department of Agriculture, Agricultural Research Service.

[21] Berger, D., et al., *Efficacy of Vitex agnus castus L. extract Ze 440 in patients with pre-menstrual syndrome (PMS).* Archives of Gynecology and Obstetrics, 2000. **264**(3): p. 150-3.

[22] Lauritzen, C., H. D. Reuter, R. Repges, K.-J. Bohnert and U. Schmidt (1997). "Treatment of premenstrual tension syndrome with Vitex agnus castus. Controlled, double-blind study versus pyridoxine." Phytomedicine **4**(3): 183-189.

[23] Milewicz, A., et al., *[Vitex agnus castus extract in the treatment of luteal phase defects due to latent hyperprolactinemia. Results of a randomized placebo-controlled double-blind study].* Arzneimittel-Forschung, 1993. **43**(7): p. 752-6.

[24] Loch, E. G., H. Selle and N. Boblitz (2000). "Treatment of premenstrual syndrome with a phytopharmaceutical formulation containing Vitex agnus castus." Journal of Womens Health & Gender-Based Medicine. **9**(3): 315-20

[25] Sliutz, G., P. Speiser, A. M. Schultz, J. Spona and R. Zeillinger (1993). "Agnus castus extracts inhibit prolactin secretion of rat pituitary cells." Hormone and Metabolic Research **25**(5): 253-5.

[26] Jarry, H., S. Leonhardt, C. Gorkow and W. Wuttke (1994). "In vitro prolactin but not LH and FSH release is inhibited by compounds in extracts of Agnus castus: direct evidence for a dopaminergic principle by the dopamine receptor assay." Experimental and Clinical Endo. **102**(6): 448-54.

www.ingramcontent.com/pod-product-compliance
Lightning Source LLC
Chambersburg PA
CBHW081419270326

41931CB00015B/3338